MANAGED CARE:
INTEGRATING THE DELIVERY AND FINANCING OF HEALTH CARE

PART C

The Health Insurance Association of America
Washington, DC 20004-1109

ISBN 1-879143-46-1

TABLE OF CONTENTS

FIGURES AND TABLES

CHAPTER 1

CHAPTER 6

CHAPTER 7

CHAPTER 8

CHAPTER 9

CHAPTER 10

FOREWORD

The HIAA Insurance Education Program aims to be the leader in providing the highest quality educational material and service to the health insurance industry and other related health care fields.

To accomplish this mission, the Program seeks to fulfill the following goals:

1. Provide a tool for use by member company personnel to enhance quality and efficiency of services to the public;
2. Provide a career development vehicle for employees and other health care industry personnel; and
3. Further general understanding of the role and contribution of the health insurance industry to the financing, administration, and delivery of health care services.

The Insurance Education Program provides the following services:

1. A comprehensive course of study in the Fundamentals of Health Insurance, Medical Expense Insurance, Disability Income Insurance, Supplemental Health Insurance, Long-Term Care Insurance, Health Insurance Fraud, and Managed Care;
2. Certification by examination of educational achievement for all courses;
3. Programs to recognize accomplishment in the industry and academic communities through course evaluation and certification, which enables participants to obtain academic or continuing education credits; and
4. Development of educational, instructional, training, and information materials related to the health insurance and health care industries.

PREFACE

Over the past 40 years, the health and disability insurance industry has undergone many profound changes. As these changes have occurred, the HIAA Insurance Education Program has sought to incorporate them into its curriculum to achieve its mission of maintaining high-quality educational material and service.

Managed care's integration of the administration and financing of health benefits with the delivery of health care services continues to significantly affect the health insurance industry. The importance of managed care has warranted the development of new HIAA Education Program curriculum materials. This text, with its accompanying self-study manual, is the latest in a series of HIAA texts on managed care.

Successful completion of the Managed Care curriculum (Parts A, B, and C), in addition to HIAA's courses in the Fundamentals of Health Insurance Part A and Part B, and Medical Expense Insurance, will lead to the HIAA designation of Managed Healthcare Professional (MHP).

Many of the concepts contained in the Managed Care curriculum are constantly in flux. Characteristics evolve over time, and insurers and managed care organizations find themselves at different stages along a continuum of managed care programs. In addition, the insurance industry operates in an ever-changing regulatory climate. These realities are important to keep in mind during the study of HIAA's entire curricula.

The contents of this book are educational, not a statement of policy. The views expressed or suggested in this and all other HIAA textbooks are those of the contributing authors or editors. They are not necessarily the opinions of HIAA or of its member companies.

ACKNOWLEDGMENTS

Chapter 1: Managed Care and the Restructuring of Health Care for Americans in the 1990s: An Overview
Russ C. Coile, Jr.
Chi Systems/Superior Consultant

Chapter 2: Managed Care and the Regulatory Arena
Thomas G. Goddard
Consultant

Chapter 3: Managed Care and the Consumer
John K. Mills
HIP Health Plans

Chapter 4: Managed Care and Public and Private Purchasing Groups
Andrea B. Castell
Castell & Associates

Chapter 5: The Federal Employees Health Benefits Program
Erling Hansen
George Washington University Health Plan

Chapter 6: TRICARE: A Managed Care Option
Jane Galvin
Health Insurance Association of America

Chapter 7: Managed Care in Medicare
Jane Galvin
Health Insurance Association of America

Chapter 8: State Government as a Purchaser of Managed Care
Lee Partridge
American Public Human Services Association

Chapter 9: Pharmacy Benefit Management Programs
Michael A. Nameth, R.Ph.
WellPoint Pharmacy Management

Chapter 10: Managed Dental Care
>Donald S. Mayes, DDS
>Don Mayes & Associates
>
>Thomas A. Dzuryachko
>United Concordia Companies, Inc.

Chapter 11: Behavioral Health Programs
>Daniel Lieberman, MD
>Value/Options Behavioral Health

Chapter 12: Vision Care Programs
>Andrew Alcorn and Stephanie Lucas
>Block Vision, Inc.

Chapter 13: Managed Care and the Physician Today
>Robert A. Berenson, M.D.
>Center for Health Plans and Providers (CHPP), Health Care Financing
>Administration

Chapter 14: Measuring and Managing the Quality of Care
>Victor G. Villagra, M.D.
>CIGNA HealthCare

Chapter 15: Managing Market-Driven Organizational Change
>Peter Boland, Ph.D.
>Boland Healthcare, Inc.

Reviewers
>Elizabeth Hoy
>Polaris Consulting
>
>Lynn Shapiro Snyder
>Epstein, Becker & Green

Editors
>Julie L. Hopkins
>Interis
>
>Tom Casacky
>Interis

ABOUT THE AUTHORS

Andrew Alcorn is Executive Vice President of Block Vision, Inc., a national vision benefits manager. He shares responsibility for strategic planning and overall performance, and oversees business development and administrative operations. Mr. Alcorn, an attorney, served as outside legal counsel before joining the company's executive management team in 1993.

Robert A. Berenson is Director of the Center for Health Plans and Providers (CHPP) in the Health Care Financing Administration. He has served on many panels and committees related to managed care and is currently chair of the Managed Care Panel on Health Care Quality of the Institute of Medicine. His extensive background in managed care includes experience as founder and medical director of a PPO and acting CEO of an HMO. Dr. Berenson is a board-certified internist and a Fellow in the American College of Physicians.

Peter Boland, Ph.D., is a well-known health care speaker and author with extensive experience in managed care. He works with many managed care organizations that seek to change to his results-oriented approach from conventional strategies and approaches. He is President of Boland Healthcare, Inc., a management consulting firm. His most recent publications include *The Capitation Sourcebook* and *Redesigning Healthcare Delivery*.

Andrea B. Castell is Managing Partner of Castell & Associates, specializing in cost and quality measurement and health system communication and information for employers and health care groups. Previously, she was Executive Director of the Health Care Purchasers Association (HCPA), where she represented the collective health care interests of employers in Washington State's business group on health. She is a past member of the Board of the National Business Coalition on Health and currently serves on the Advisory Council for the State of Washington Basic Health Plan (BHP) and on the editorial board of *Business and Health* magazine.

Russ C. Coile, Jr., is Senior Vice President of Chi Systems/Superior Consultant, a health care strategy and management consulting firm. Mr. Coile is a recognized health care futurist. He is editor of *Russ Coile's Health Trends*, a monthly newsletter, and has authored five books on the future of health care, most recently *The Five Stages of Managed Care*.

Thomas A. Dzuryachko is President of United Concordia Companies, Inc. (UCCI), a national dental insurance company. He was instrumental in creating UCCI from the Pennsylvania Blue Shield dental program in 1992. His experience includes senior positions in marketing and finance for the Blue Cross and Blue Shield plans in Pennsylvania.

Jane Galvin is Director of Managed Care Policy for the Health Insurance Association of America, where she is the issue manager for managed care issues related to federal and state legislative and regulatory issues. Her career includes 20 years with Kaiser Permanente Mid-Atlantic, where she was responsible for state and federal regulatory activities in the region, and for policy development and benefit issues. Ms. Galvin also worked as a congressional staffer within the House of Representatives and for the Group Health Association of America (now the American Association of Health Plans).

Thomas Goddard is an attorney who consults on health care management and public policy. Most recently, he was Vice President and Regional General Counsel for NYLCare Health Plans of the Mid-Atlantic, Inc., where he was responsible for legal, legislative, and regulatory affairs. He also has worked for the National Association of Insurance Commissioners, the Goddard Public Affairs Corporation, the Alliance for Consumer Rights, the Association of Trial Lawyers of America, and then-Arizona Governor Bruce Babbitt. Mr. Goddard is completing his Ph.D. in industrial-organizational psychology at George Mason University.

Erling Hansen is Director of Legal and Regulatory Affairs for the George Washington University Health Plan, a federally qualified HMO participating in the FEHB Program. An attorney, Mr. Hansen served as General Counsel of the American Association of Health Plans from 1979 to 1994. He also worked for the U.S. Civil Service Commission as a contracting official in the FEHB Program and as editor of *HMO Law Manual,* published by Aspen Systems Corporation.

Daniel Lieberman is Regional Medical Director for Value/Options Behavioral Health. He has 10 years' experience as senior medical director and executive manager with two of the largest national behavioral health care organizations. For the National Committee for Quality Assurance (NCQA), he serves as a surveyor and a member of both its MBHO Scoring Task Force and its planning committee for training. He is board-certified in child/adolescent psychiatry and adult psychiatry and maintains a private practice in New York City.

Stephanie Lucas has over 10 years' experience in managed health care. Currently she is Vice President, Administration, for Block Vision, Inc., and is responsible for account implementation and management, CQI, and marketing. Ms. Lucas is a Certified Professional in Healthcare Quality and holds a master's degree in business administration.

Michael A. Nameth, R.Ph., is General Manager of WellPoint Pharmacy Management, where he has responsibility for all pharmacy operations, including clinical programs, pharmacy network contracting, claims processing, and customer service. He has overseen design and implementation of WellPoint's online, on-demand pharmacy system and its proprietary Maximum Allowable Cost program. Mr. Nameth has 15 years' experience in pharmacy practice in managed care and was Director of Pharmacy Services for Blue Cross Blue Shield plans in Michigan and Cincinnati.

Donald S. Mayes is a dentist and the Principal of Don Mayes & Associates, a dental benefits consulting firm. He is author of numerous articles on dental benefits that have appeared in the *Wall Street Journal*, *Money* magazine, and many trade journals. His book, *Managed Dental Care: A Guide to Dental HMOs*, is in its fourth printing. His experience includes senior management positions in dental benefits for major insurance and third-party administrators. He is a Fellow in the American College of Medical Quality and the Academy of Dentistry International.

John K. Mills is Director of Federal Relations for HIP Health Plans. Prior to joining HIP in 1995, Mr. Mills was the Legislative Director to Representative Eliot L. Engel of New York, where he worked on health care and ERISA issues and served on the President's Task Force on Health Care Reform.

Lee Partridge has more than 20 years' experience with state health insurance programs, including oversight responsibility as chief of staff for a state legislative committee and nine years as state Medicaid director. Currently she is Director of the Health Policy unit of the American Public Human Services Organization (formerly the American Public Welfare Association), and works on a daily basis with state Medicaid and child health insurance program administrators across the country.

Victor G. Villagra is Vice President of Quality and Care Management at CIGNA HealthCare (CHC), where he is responsible for strategic planning and oversight of all national quality improvement initiatives, including health plan accreditation, credentialing, and disease management programs. He heads CHC's Technology Assessment Council and its Health Promotion/Disease Prevention Council. Prior to joining CIGNA, he was Medical Director of Geisinger Continuous Health Improvement Program. Dr. Villagra is a board-certified internist and a Fellow of the American College of Physicians.

Section I

THE STATE OF MANAGED CARE

Significant changes in managed care began to occur in 1996, and continue in 1998. During this period, managed care experienced rapid growth, becoming the market-share leader in many parts of the country. This growth has been accompanied by a barrage of criticism from consumers and providers that has been echoed in the media, prompting an outpouring of legislation at federal and state levels. In response, managed care organizations initiated new products, expanded provider networks, and consolidated. This book builds on the foundation established in Parts A and B by presenting what is new or changed in managed care and by identifying the key trends and issues that MCOs must address to remain successful.

Managed Care: Integrating the Delivery and Financing of Health Care Part C addresses these changes and the alterations that will be required—both industrywide and by individual MCOs—if their success is to continue. This initial section updates the description of the state of managed care today. Chapter 1 identifies the overall trends, growth, and issues reshaping the industry. Chapter 2 reviews new or proposed federal and state legislation that burdens MCOs with additional costs and potentially stifles industry-sponsored innovations. Chapter 3 defines consumers' issues with managed care, discusses the focus of media attention on these issues, and explains how consumers (who generally are not direct purchasers of care) influence legislation, employer purchasing decisions, and MCO products.

Chapter 1

MANAGED CARE AND THE RESTRUCTURING OF HEALTH CARE FOR AMERICANS IN THE 1990s: AN OVERVIEW

■ Introduction

Managed care made great strides in recent years, emerging in the mid-1990s as America's market-oriented approach to health reform. Rejecting the health care plan proposed by President Clinton, the nation's employers and consumers turned to managed care organizations (MCOs) as the solution to rising health care costs. As of July 1, 1996, more than 63 million Americans (representing one in four health care consumers of all types) were enrolled in managed care plans. The numbers are growing steadily, at an annual rate of 18.7 percent. Regions like the Southeast, initially slow to accept managed care, saw a 19.4 percent growth rate in MCO membership in 1996–1997.[1] Enrollment in managed health care plans is likely to top 100 million within five years, spurred by Congress's support for Medicare and Medicaid MCOs in its 1997 budget reform legislation.

This growth represents a considerable change from "the old days" when health maintenance organizations (HMOs)—an early form of MCO—were innovative new models that challenged a well-entrenched health insurance industry. Called "prepaid practice plans" or "alternative delivery systems," the HMOs were supported with federal grants and regulatory protection from the established indemnity health insurers. The rising acceptance of managed care and its cost controls accelerated the movement away from traditional indemnity insurance. Managed care's approach reduced the utilization of hospitals and ancillary

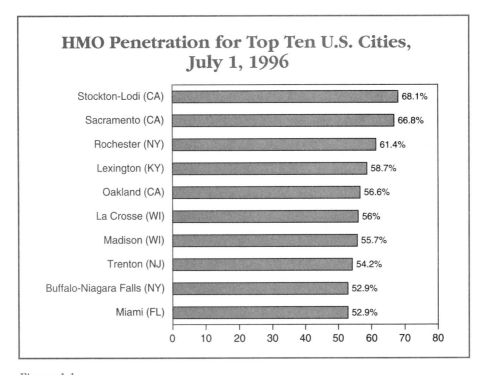

HMO Penetration for Top Ten U.S. Cities, July 1, 1996

City	Penetration
Stockton-Lodi (CA)	68.1%
Sacramento (CA)	66.8%
Rochester (NY)	61.4%
Lexington (KY)	58.7%
Oakland (CA)	56.6%
La Crosse (WI)	56%
Madison (WI)	55.7%
Trenton (NJ)	54.2%
Buffalo-Niagara Falls (NY)	52.9%
Miami (FL)	52.9%

Figure 1.1

SOURCE: Hamer, R. 1997. "HMO Regional Market Analysis." Part III. July, p. 4.

services, decreased excess testing, and brought health inflation rates below the consumer price index.

Market Penetration

Initially, skeptics predicted that managed care could never gain more than a limited share of any local market. Now, there are 10 cities across the United States with greater than 50 percent managed care enrollment (see Figure 1.1). It is not surprising that three high-penetration cities are located in California, a leader in managed care, but the list also includes markets as diverse as Lexington, Buffalo, and Miami. The popularity of managed care with government workers partly explains the penetration in the three cities that are also state capitals: Sacramento, Madison, and Trenton.

At a local level, a pattern of dominance emerges in which three or four of the largest MCOs hold 60–75 percent of the market.[2] Every market differs, and the top MCOs in a market are not always national firms. For example:

- In the Dallas-Fort Worth (TX) market, a provider-sponsored plan, Harris Methodist, is the leader.
- Three local MCOs, including Kaiser, PacifiCare/FHP, and Foundation Health, dominate California.
- Blue Cross-owned HMOs are the top plans in a number of markets, including Portland (OR), Cleveland (OH), and Pittsburgh (PA). As a result of their hesitancy to enter the managed care market, Blue Cross/Blue Shield plans are only second-tier players in other regions.

In the largest metropolitan areas (more than one million population), the market is typically distributed as follows:

- the leader holds a 38 percent market share;
- the number two plan holds a 21 percent share;
- the number three plan holds a 12 percent share; and
- the remaining 29 percent is divided among as many as 15–20 other MCOs.[3]

Mid-sized markets (populations of 250,000 to one million) are more concentrated, with the leader commanding a 53 percent share. Small markets (under 250,000) are the least competitive: The leading health plan typically maintains a 69 percent share and the numbers two through four plans split 31 percent of the local enrollment.

In 1996, HMO membership fell by 3–5 percent, and sometimes more, in a number of markets, including Albany (NY), Bergen-Passaic (NJ), Boston (MA), Cleveland (OH), Gary (IN), Los Angeles (CA), Nassau-Suffolk (NY), and Worcester (MA). The drop in enrollment reflects, in part, those consumers who are "buying up" to obtain greater access and choice by switching to preferred provider organizations (PPOs) . Some market observers believe the MCO movement is "running out of steam." That could happen, argues Dr. Jerome Kassirer, unless managed care plans "show that they have become better citizens: that they care about more than profits, that they don't skimp on care, that they support their share of teaching, research and care of the poor, that they no longer muzzle physicians, and that they offer something special (including control of costs) by managing care."[4]

New Competition for Market Share

Nearly 40 new MCOs emerged between 1993 and 1998, many of which were created by providers. Physicians and hospitals are launching provider-sponsored plans, especially in markets with less than 25 percent managed care penetration. However, even in mature markets (for example, Minneapolis, with its high managed care penetration), provider-sponsored plans gain market share as em-ployers—looking for ways to reduce costs and to provide employees with more choice—bypass the HMOs.

Medical societies joined in the managed care competition, but most of these physician-backed efforts grow slowly. For example, the MCO owned by the California Medical Association (CMA) attracted more physicians than enrollees in its statewide network. In June 1998, CMA announced a plan to end its managed care business.

■ The Maturing Managed Care Marketplace

A national survey of more than 2,000 firms indicated that more than 80 percent of U.S. workers with health insurance (not including those on Medicare, Medi-caid, etc.) now receive their coverage through some form of MCO—an HMO, PPO, or point-of-service (POS) plan. Managed care plans are now commonplace in small firms as well as large ones. Typically, small companies offer only one health plan. In the past, it was an indemnity plan or PPO, but today it is more likely to be an HMO or PPO plan. Even government-sponsored beneficiaries opt for managed care plans. By the turn of the century, managed care growth will have occurred in dozens of states beyond the five core markets (California, New York, Florida, Oregon, and Massachusetts).

Managed Care Growth and Trends by Purchaser

In purchasing health care coverage, the nation's consumers are moving toward a middle or "lite" version of managed care from two extremes: traditional HMOs (gatekeeper model) and traditional indemnity (non-managed) plans. Potentially, the greatest changes will affect managed care plans for government beneficiaries. The conversion of Medicare and Medicaid eligibles (who account for less than 25 percent of the population, but 40 percent of health care spend-ing) into managed care coverage is one of the "megatrends" in health care. Em-ployers continue to be major purchasers of managed care, with significant growth in the small employer (offering employees one health plan) sector.

Medicare

The number of Medicare-related managed care reforms enacted by Congress in mid-1997 could drive Medicare HMO penetration from 10 percent in 1997 to 20–25 percent by 2003. The enrollment of seniors in Medicare HMOs climbed at double-digit rates between 1992 and 1997, jumping 35.5 percent in 1996.[5] Congress's far-reaching reforms include raising the floor of Medicare HMO payments to $350 per member/per month, eliminating the 1:1 requirement to balance seniors with commercial HMO enrollees, and creating PPO and provider-sponsored organization (PSO) options. Those changes should expand managed care in rural areas, where Medicare HMO fees are below cost under the old scheme of Medicare HMO payments. Younger and healthier seniors, aged 65–75, are likely to sign up first. The projections for older seniors, above age 75, are more cautionary, given the resistance shown toward switching to managed care, even if an individual can save $1,000 or more by dropping supplemental "Medi-gap" coverage.[6]

Medicaid

Because of the predictable costs of managed care programs, states are implementing them as the means to provide medical care to Medicaid beneficiaries. Through managed care, state governments shift the management responsibility (as well as the economic risk) to capitated plans and provider networks. Beginning in 1993, Medicaid capitation soared at annual rates between 22 percent and 42 percent, reaching 57.6 percent growth in 1996. Nearly 20 states have converted to capitation. Another 18 states (including New York, with the largest Medicaid program in the nation) have submitted waiver requests to the Health Care Financing Administration (HCFA). New York and California have already shifted more than 400,000 Medicaid beneficiaries into managed care. Medicaid HMOs are capitalizing on the opportunity. The top 25 Medicaid HMOs have between 50,000 and 250,000 enrollees. By 2000, Medicaid HMOs may be the dominant Medicaid option in more than 40 states.[7]

Employer Coalitions

The imprint of employer coalitions and business groups on the future of health care delivery is far from clear. To date, their impact has been limited. Although more than 100 business coalitions focus on health care, few take advantage of their clout in the market (e.g., through group purchasing). Some notable exceptions are:

- Buyers Health Care Action Group in Minnesota, with its innovative model of direct contracting with 24 local provider-sponsored networks;[8]
- San Francisco's Pacific Business Group on Health (PBGH), which pressured California HMOs to substantially reduce premiums. PBGH offers incentives to HMOs to improve customer satisfaction and health promotion by withholding a portion of the premium unless goals are met.

More direct contracting may occur in rural areas, where employers are offered fewer managed care choices. In Statesboro, Georgia, near Savannah, a 36-member coalition pooled its health care clout and saved $41 million by contracting with local physician-hospital organizations.[9] If by 2001 MCOs raise prices beyond the consumer price index, employer coalitions may look into either collective purchasing or direct contracting.

Self-Funded Employers (ERISA)

Congress is eroding the protection of employer-sponsored plans granted under the federal Employee Retirement Income Security Act (ERISA). The 1996 enactment of the Health Insurance Portability and Accountability Act (HIPAA) required employers with ERISA plans to provide "parity" between mental health and other health benefits. As a result, some employers dropped their mental health coverage. ERISA protection was also weakened by the courts. A Texas federal judge recently validated a state-enacted "any willing provider" law against ERISA plans, forcing employer self-funded plans to open their pharmacy networks to competing pharmacies. In the future, large self-funded employers may shift strategies and return to the commercial insurance market, most likely to buy managed care plans.

Small Employers

Although many small employers remain uninsured, firms with fewer than 50 employees that do provide health coverage are switching to managed care plans. Sixty-nine percent of employees[10] working in these small firms were enrolled in managed care plans in 1995, up dramatically from 22 percent in 1993. With HIPAA, prices for small employers declined when plans were required to guarantee coverage to any member of an enrolled group, regardless of his/her current or past health status. In many markets, the local chambers of commerce formed health care pools to purchase managed care coverage for small businesses. By 2000, an estimated 80 percent of the individual and small group market will purchase managed care plans.[11]

Market Growth and Trends by Type of Plan

Changes in the demographics of purchasers of health care, rapid growth, and a competitive marketplace forced changes in the products offered by MCOs. Initial success resulted from price competition; now, managed care organizations must present a more varied portfolio. Doing so can be a business advantage, because some new products carry higher prices and profit margins. MCO product lines are also reshaped, as more consumer-friendly options (POS, open access, and PPO) gain market share against conventional HMOs and the rapidly disappearing indemnity plans. By one industry estimate, the number of PPO

Table 1.1

"Lite" Managed Care Products Will Increase Market Share

	Percentage increase of privately insured	
Type of plan	1997	2000
Indemnity	37	20
PPO	25	40
Point-of-service (POS)	15	20
HMO	23	20

SOURCE: Peter W. Nauert, "Managed Care: A Year 2000 Design," *National Underwriter,* Life & Health Edition, April 28, 1997, p. 14.

and POS plans is expected to exceed the number of HMO and indemnity plans by the year 2000 (see Table 1.1).

Commercial HMOs

In advanced managed care markets like Southern California and Minnesota, aggressive pricing strategies in the mid-1990s pushed managed care prices into the $90–$95 per member/per month range (or even lower). The counter trend is for MCOs to boost prices and offer easier access to specialists and alternative medicine as incentives for consumers to purchase a premium-priced product. Many markets remain price-competitive, but lower stock prices for publicly traded MCOs may contribute to higher premiums. As HMO premiums rise between 1998 and 2001, employers may turn to cost-competitive alternatives, such as direct provider contracting.

POS (Point-of-Service) Plans

According to estimates by KPMG Peat Marwick, POS plans accounted for 20.1 percent of the market in 1997, significantly more than double their 9.1 percent share in 1993.[12] In the mid-Atlantic states, where 38 percent of the nation's 6.2 million POS enrollees reside, POS plans outsell HMOs by 2:1. The phenomenal growth of POS plans demonstrates the popularity of "lite" managed care, whereby enrollees are given more choices and partial coverage if they use out-of-network health services. Most POS enrollees (80 percent) are enrolled in larger managed care plans (more than 50,000 members). Consumers, or their employers, are willing to pay premiums that average 8–12 percent higher than traditional HMO plans. In the future, other "lite" managed care options, such as the open-access product, may offer a lower-cost alternative to POS plans, yet respond to consumer demands for greater access to specialists.

Open-access Plans

Like the POS plan, open-access arrangements allow patients to bypass their gate-keepers and seek specialty medical care, but only within the MCO's provider network. To hedge against the costs of higher utilization, the open-access plan imposes a surcharge for the privilege of self-referral—typically a $15–$25 copayment at the time of service. Prices for open-access products run a modest 5–8 percent above traditional HMO premiums. As a consumer-friendly variation of the network HMO model, open-access plans present an attractive option to indemnity or PPO enrollees who want more choices but lower premiums.

PPOs (Preferred Provider Organizations)

Preferred provider organizations (PPOs) represent the future for today's commercial indemnity plans. PPOs offer consumers a choice of providers at prices below managed indemnity plans. They are popular with consumers but more expensive—typically 15–25 percent higher than HMO plans.[13] In general, PPOs are popular among fee-for-service medical providers because there are few limitations on the amount of services they can provide; the trade-off is that medical providers in PPOs must keep their charges low. PPOs will continue to be a viable managed care product if prices remain affordable for the average consumer.

Managed Indemnity Plans

Traditional (unmanaged) indemnity health insurance has been replaced by managed indemnity plans, which offer unlimited provider choices but with higher deductibles. Indemnity plans are priced 25–40 percent higher than MCOs in the same market. Managed indemnity plans insist on prior authorization for expensive services and may deny claims for services that the plans consider medically unnecessary. Managed indemnity may become obsolete, because of its lack of effective cost controls and high prices. Few companies cover more than 80 percent of the costs of benefits, and many fix their employer contribution to the HMO premiums, effectively making indemnity a very expensive choice for consumers. By 2005 (or sooner), indemnity plans are likely to fall below 10 percent of national market share and be replaced by less expensive PPO and POS plans.

Medical Savings Accounts

New to the market, Medical Savings Accounts (MSAs) are an innovative insurance product. A form of indemnity insurance, MSAs combine a high-deductible insurance policy with a savings account.[14] The savings from a higher deductible goes to an MSA account to cover routine medical expenses, while the high-deductible insurance plan covers expenses that exceed the deductible. At year-end the consumer keeps whatever remains in his or her Medical Savings Account. HIPAA authorized up to 400,000 people (who are self-employed or in small companies with a maximum of 50 workers) to participate in a four-year pilot test of MSAs. In 1997, Congress allowed a limited number of Medi-care-eligibles to enroll in MSAs. Enrollment has been slow: The total number of MSA enrollees was less than 50,000 by mid-1997. The slow start has been attrib-uted to "market inertia" and to the disruption to employer benefit plans caused by the addition of an MSA option.[15] Some employers express their concern that MSAs encourage employees to delay seeking care until a health condition be-comes a major (and costly) problem. Unless adopted by a substantial number of large, self-insured employers, the MSA option is unlikely to be successful.

■ Issues in the Managed Care Marketplace

MCOs are winning market share, but often at the expense of heavy criticism from consumer groups. Managed care's economic focus provokes consumer and provider resentment, which is often presented in the media. Providers view managed care's controls over utilization and treatment authorization as ar-bitrary. Their views are expressed by the American Medical Association's (AMA) model legislation—the "Patient Protection Act"—which was used by a number of state legislatures to enact managed care reform bills. In another example of resistance, physicians in California formed a union and recruited 20 percent of the state's 70,000 doctors.[16] To increase their bargaining clout, the doctors' union joined the AFL-CIO's American Federation of State, County, and Munici-pal Employees.

Government Regulation

Not long ago, HMOs were the underdogs and state legislation was necessary to protect them from the powerful insurance companies. Times have changed. Legislators now respond to consumers, providers, and the media, who are united in their criticism of managed care. In 1996 alone, more than 1,000 bills that addressed consumer concerns about managed care were introduced in state legislatures and Congress,[17] and hundreds of such bills have since become law. Some typical laws passed by different states include the following:

- providers who are under incentive clauses to limit care must disclose finan-cial conflicts of interest;
- gag rules, which prohibited physicians from criticizing plans or fully inform-ing patients about treatment, are prohibited;

- physicians, hospitals, chiropractors, pharmacies, and others cannot be shut out of HMO contracts if the providers are willing to accept HMO prices and terms ("any willing provider" laws);

- consumers are guaranteed choice-of-plan options;

- in Texas, managed care plans are specifically identified as potentially liable for denials of treatment; and

- HMOs and insurers cannot arbitrarily drop a provider from a network without a fair hearing (i.e., due process).

HIPAA moved managed care reform to the national level by guaranteeing the right of at least a 48-hour stay for maternity admissions and imposing mental health parity on health plans with more than 50 employees. Congress expanded access to MSAs and private health care in the 1997 budget deficit reform legislation. During the same year, the Clinton administration used executive orders to guarantee certain patient rights under Medicare and Medicaid HMOs. More reform of managed care is expected: President Clinton's Advisory Commission on Consumer Protection and Quality in the Health Care Industry, which in 1997 issued a patient's rights list, recommended further managed care reform legislation in its final report.

Competition and Profits

After three years of competitive pricing and growing market share, in 1998 many MCOs raised their premiums to improve profit margins, even if doing so meant the loss of double-digit enrollment growth. Across the industry, the market experience had been the same: Enrollments rose but profits for a number of MCOs declined (see Table 1.2). In 1996, MCO membership rose an average of 19.2 percent among large, publicly traded managed care plans. However, profits fell to a scant 0.2 percent for year-end, after two years of widespread price competition hurt earnings.[18] Lower profits continued into 1997, with the managed care industry running operating losses of 0.3 percent in the first quarter of 1997, despite 3-4 percent higher premiums imposed on January 1. Wall Street took its toll on publicly traded MCOs, slashing stock prices by 20-30 percent, where their shares languished at the end of 1997. However, with hopes that double-digit rate increases for 1998 will bolster profits, investors sent the price of MCO stocks soaring (up over 35 percent in the first five months of that year).

Price competition among managed care plans was a major factor in the de-escalation of health costs in the 1990s. By the mid-1990s, the rate of health care expenditures slowed below the annual rate of consumer inflation, then

Table 1.2

Profit Margins in Leading, Publicly Traded HMOs

National HMOs	Revenues*		Net income*		Total enrollments	
	1996	1995	1996	1995	1996	1995
United Healthcare Corporation	10,074.0	5,671.0	356.0	286.0	13,778,000	3,653,000
Aetna U.S. Healthcare	7,765.2	5,949.7	58.7	286.0	14,210,000	14,396,000
Humana Inc.	6,788.0	4,702.0	12.0	190.0	4,851,000	3,804,400
Wellpoint Health Networks	4,170.0	3,107.1	202.0	180.0	4,484,701	2,797,362
Oxford Health Plans	3,075.0	1,765.4	99.6	52.4	1,535,000	1,007,700
Healthsource	1,714.0	1,167.0	(3.9)	56.3	3,172,800	3,426,100
PacifiCare Health Systems	1,134.0	1,064.3	32.0	28.0	2,045,109	1,816,432
MidAtlantic Medical	1,134.0	955.0	(2.8)	61.1	1,679,600	1,483,400
Coventry Corporation	1,057.1	852.4	(61.3)	.018	901,891	780,775

* In millions
SOURCE: Niedzielski, J. "HMOs Hike Premiums After So-So '96." *National Underwriter*, Life & Health Edition, Mar. 17, 1997, p. 1.

began to rise slowly as MCOs raised premiums. The high volume of health plans, with 15–20 MCOs competing in many large metropolitan areas, continues to fuel a competitive market. Even when large-scale consolidation occurs, both large and small plans are often forced to compete on price. The largest MCOs can "buy the market" with low premiums that are aimed at driving smaller competitors out of a market. Fighting back, small plans compete on price but must differentiate their offerings from those of the "big plans" through better consumer service. This scenario could remain the same for the rest of the 1990s if price competition limits premium increases to a moderate 2–5 percent annually. However, many health plans sought to further strengthen profits and share prices by proposing double-digit rate increases in 1998. Nonprofit plans joined the trend: Kaiser Permanente, for example, sought a 12 percent rate increase. In Minneapolis, the three large managed care companies raised premiums as much as 15 percent. Small employers were especially hard hit, with premium increases of more than 40 percent. If MCOs try to regain high-level profits too quickly, they could open the door for direct-provider contracting and increase the competition from provider-sponsored MCOs.

Increases in premiums point to the managed care industry's limited ability to control medical costs. The industry's average medical loss ratio increased to 84.3 percent in 1996, up from 81.9 percent the previous year. MCOs struggle to contain rising medical claims, especially for pharmacy and outpatient care. Only in California, where medical loss ratios rose a minimal 0.8 percent, have MCOs been successful in holding the line on medical expenses.

13

Industry Consolidation

Beginning in 1997, MCOs began a consolidation trend. These mergers resulted from the hope that larger organizations could dominate a market. The 10 largest plans now account for 45.2 percent of all managed care enrollees.[19] Health plans affiliated with national firms, including Blue Cross/Blue Shield, account for 79.9 percent—more than 50 million—of all managed care members. Recent mergers included:

- CIGNA and HealthSource

- PacifiCare and FHP

- Foundation Health and Health Systems International

- WellPoint and John Hancock

- Aetna U.S. Healthcare and NYLCare

Large firms, such as United Healthcare, completed a number of smaller deals to enter new markets and build market share. Smaller plans hope to improve a marginal market position through a merger, or to rescue a marginal financial situation by consolidation with a larger "white knight."

Provider-Sponsored MCOs

Despite the concentration of market power in larger firms, new provider-sponsored MCOs continue to emerge. Consolidation of providers into more than 500 regional networks has put physicians and hospitals in a position to compete for—and potentially control—the premium. Provider-sponsored MCOs that lack critical mass or break-even potential may try to consolidate with commercial plans in order to gain access to capital, management expertise, and infrastructure. In 1997, a number of provider-sponsored plans were sold or entered into joint ventures

- Chicago's Advocate Health System recently sold its HMO to Humana under a 10-year preferred provider agreement.

- In Seattle, the Virginia Mason Health Plan has been sold to Aetna U.S. Healthcare, which once owned 20 percent of the provider-owned plan.[20] The deal will reunite Aetna and the Virginia Mason Medical Center, joining to compete against the affiliation of rival Group Health Plan of Puget Sound with Kaiser Permanente/Oregon.

Enactment of PSO legislation authorized the federal HCFA to contract with providers to serve Medicare beneficiaries, with a three-year waiver from state licensing requirements. States may choose to license PSOs and thus open the door for providers to participate in Medicaid-risk programs at the state level.

▓ MCOs' Responses Determine Success or Failure

To continue to succeed, MCOs must rearrange their business strategies in the following ways:

Be Consumer-Driven

Respond to consumers' requests for user-friendly care with innovative, "out-of-the-box" programs and products.

Simplify Access and Increase Choices

Enhance service image by reducing treatment authorization red tape and expanding provider networks to increase choices for the consumer.

Remain Price-Competitive

Stay price-competitive (otherwise, employers may decide to contract directly with delivery systems).

Promote Clinically Efficient Processes

Concentrate on the 80 percent cost factor—the medical loss ratio—to improve medical efficiency with better clinical processes for early diagnosis and prompt and effective treatment.

Reduce Overhead

Lower administrative expenses. Purchasers won't tolerate plans that spend too high a percentage of the premium on administration before delivering any medical care.

Establish Provider Alliances

Create long-term strategic business alliances with regional provider networks. MCOs must recognize that providers are essential to customer satisfaction and should seek alliances with well-known providers.

Demonstrate Value to Purchasers

Show employers and government purchasers that the MCO's plan "adds value" through lower administrative expenses, a higher medical loss ratio, health promotion, customer service, and clinical outcomes.

Accept Accountability

Meet employer and government demands for accountability by issuing "report cards" for costs and health status. Focus attention on improving the health status of large, capitated populations.

■ Challenges for Managed Care

To survive in the next century, MCOs must progress even beyond the recommendations above and reinvent themselves. Growth and market consolidation, greater consumer choice, and more savvy public relations are insufficient to meet the major challenge of the 21st century: managing the health needs of an expanding, aging population. To answer this challenge, MCOs must address several critical factors.

1. Population Health Management

The largest challenge immediately facing health care in the next century is to manage the health risks and costs of an aging population. As more elderly and high-risk individuals enroll in health plans, and underwriting is restricted by health reform, actual differences in health plan performance will be required to generate savings for the customer and earnings for the MCO.[21] Health plans with foresight are gearing up to serve millions of chronically ill enrollees through full-risk arrangements under Medicare.

2. Public Health Partnership

An MCO's interest in public health problems rises when it becomes responsible for providing care to the poor (Medicaid) and the elderly (Medicare). Innovative partnerships between public health agencies and managed care plans can unify public and private resources to bear on a number of key health status issues, such as:

- childhood immunizations;
- cancer screening;
- prenatal care;
- AIDS prevention;
- communicable diseases (e.g., STD, TB);
- tobacco and alcohol control; and
- consumer health education.

■ Conclusion

There are trends and counter-trends in managed care today. Overall, trends favor the domination of many markets by large national firms, with consolidation of enrollment among three to four plans in local markets.

When the dust of managed care competition settles, who will be the winners and losers? Midwest-based market observer Dr. Montague Brown argues that "Among all this change are massive struggles for power, influence and control. Who wins? Those who realize the dream of delivering best value. Who wins matters less because [hospitals, managed care companies, and physician organizations] are all moving toward integrated organizations that incorporate financing, physician services, and institutional care under one corporate and/or partnered umbrella."[22]

■ Key Terms

Employer coalitions
Employment Retirement Income Security Act (ERISA)
Health Insurance Portability and Accountability Act (HIPAA)

Managed care "lite"
Managed indemnity
Market consolidation
Medicaid managed care
Medical Savings Accounts (MSAs)
Medicare managed care
Open-access plans

Patient Protection Act
Point-of-service (POS) plans
Preferred provider organization (PPO) plans
Provider-sponsored MCO

Chapter 2

MANAGED CARE AND THE REGULATORY ARENA

■ Introduction

Compared with most modern western industrial nations, the United States minimally regulates its major industries. Yet regulation plays a dominant role in the life of most American companies. Few major industries have avoided the oversight of the Occupational Safety and Health Administration (OSHA), the Equal Employment Opportunity Commission (EEOC), the Environmental Protection Agency (EPA), or the Consumer Product Safety Commission (CPSC). The influence of these agencies and of other regulatory bodies reaches across the boundaries of all industries and is known as horizontal regulation.

Some businesses are also subject to regulatory agencies that focus solely on their industry (vertical regulation). Examples of such agencies are the Federal Communications Commission (FCC) that regulates radio and television, and the Food and Drug Administration (FDA) that oversees the manufacture and distribution of drugs.

Health care and insurance are two industries that cope with oversight by numerous horizontal and vertical regulatory agencies. Within the vertical spectrum are regulators that focus on the entire industry and others that focus on subsets—for example, managed care. The nature and history of the managed care industry produced a highly complex regulatory structure involving multiple federal agencies and multiple state agencies with occasionally competing missions and overlapping jurisdictions. That complexity has led to high levels of uncertainty for both the managed care organizations (MCOs) and the regulators themselves.

The rapid pace of change in the health care market and in the policy debates surrounding that market may quickly erode the relevance of some of the specific information that follows. However, it is likely that the general forces described below will continue for years to come.

■ Modifying the Scope of Regulatory Power

Historically, the boundary between what the states could regulate and what was reserved to the federal government by the preemptions found in the Employee Retirement Income Security Act (ERISA)[23] was defined by the phrase "regulation of the business of insurance." The states regulated the business of insurance, while most of the other employee benefits fell to the U.S. Department of Labor. Dissatisfied with limits on their regulatory authority, however, the states initiated legislative and regulatory efforts to push back that boundary.

ERISA Preemption and the Limits of State Regulatory Authority

In the early 19th century, the states began to regulate insurance companies, deriving legal authority from state corporation laws. States formed the first insurance departments in mid-century. Scattered efforts to regulate insurers coalesced in 1872 with the formation of the National Association of Insurance Commissioners (NAIC), the oldest association of state officials.

State authority to regulate insurers remained largely unchallenged until the mid-20th century. In 1944, the Supreme Court allowed Congress to enter the arena of insurance regulation. In 1945, Congress restrained itself by passing the McCarran-Ferguson Act, which reserved to the states the regulation of the "business of insurance." With the reservation of the authority grounded on nothing but congressional self-restraint, the situation can be—and has been—subjected to unilateral modification by Congress in the years since the passage of McCarran-Ferguson.

In 1970, Congress approved ERISA, which focused primarily on the pension rights of American employees. One aspect of this gargantuan bill that received little discussion at the time preempts state laws and regulations that interfere with the essential operation of health benefit plans.

The "Business of Insurance"

It is important to distinguish between the "business of insurance," which is largely the domain of state regulation, and the "business of insurers," which is not.[24] The courts look at the nature of the relationships, not the nature of the involved companies, to determine whether the activity in question is the "business of insurance." However, there is no easy way to determine whether an activity is the business of insurance. The Supreme Court set forth a test to help courts make such a determination by asking three questions:

- Does the activity have "the effect of transferring or spreading a policyholder's risk"?
- Is the activity "an integral part of the policy relationship between the insurer and the insured"?
- Is the activity "limited to entities within the insurance industry"?[25]

If the answer to all three of these questions is "yes," a court is likely to find that the activity is the "business of insurance" for purposes of the ERISA preemption. However, recent law reveals that these questions are not enough to determine whether a state law is affected by the preemption clause of ERISA; courts must also examine whether the challenged law "relates to" the business of insurance.[26] The Supreme Court has not suggested that ERISA preempts only direct regulation of ERISA plans, but it did rule that the law does not preempt regulation that has only a remote, indirect impact on ERISA plans.

■ Alternative Formulations of the Limits of State Power

The states take diverse approaches to distinguish the boundary between state and federal regulatory authority, particularly as applied to the regulation of MCOs. The particular issue raised by the regulation of MCOs relates to the fact that they often share risk with the providers of health care, including physicians, hospitals, and physician-hospital organizations (PHOs). Examples of such risk sharing include capitated payments, risk corridors, and other payment arrangements that expose the provider to some level of insurance risk.

Sometimes regulators view the providers that accept risk from MCOs as engaged in the "business of insurance" and therefore subject to state regulation. An example of the extreme version of this view occurred in 1995, when the Virginia Bureau of Insurance (VBOI) issued an administrative letter explaining that all capitation arrangements involved the transfer of risk and, thus, the business of insurance. Based on this premise, the VBOI concluded that when a third-party administrator entered into capitated arrangements with providers in a network, ERISA did not preempt the state oversight of the "insurance" aspects of that arrangement, such as the benefits offered and the forms and rates used, even when the employer retained the risk normally passed on to the MCO. Thus, it is the present view of the VBOI that there is no such thing as an ERISA-preempt self-insured health benefit plan, as long as providers are compensated through capitation arrangements.[27] No courts have yet overturned this view.

Risk-Bearing Entities Subject to Regulation

As health care financing developed, the number and variety of entities that bore insurance risk increased. Of particular importance is the rise of provider-sponsored organizations (PSOs), in which hospitals, physicians, or other health care providers create networks for the sale of health care benefits or services either directly to employer groups or to health carriers (such as HMOs or insurers).

Recognizing the public interest in protecting consumers—both from insolvency and from improper market conduct of such entities—state insurance regulators are working to modernize their regulations. The central project in this regard is the National Association of Insurance Commissioners' (NAIC) health insurance regulatory reform initiative, known as Consolidated Licensure for Entities Assuming Risk (CLEAR). The NAIC envisions that the CLEAR project will create a seamless licensure process for all entities assuming risk, no matter what the corporate structure of such entities. The NAIC is unlikely to complete this project before 2000, or even later.

An important piece of the CLEAR project involved the development of a white paper, "Regulation of Health Risk-Bearing Entities," that reviews the changing nature of the health insurance market and the states' regulatory response. This seminal paper, adopted by the NAIC in December 1997, details the various regulatory approaches taken by the states. As of May 1997, only 10 states had a separate regulatory structure for provider-sponsored organizations. This reflects (in part) the view that existing managed care laws are sufficient to sweep into the domain of state regulation any PSOs or other entities that may want to operate in the states.

However, health care provider organizations, notably hospital and physician associations, have urged legislators to ease solvency requirements for provider-sponsored networks (PSNs) that assume risk. How regulators react to those requests depends primarily on the nature of the entities from which the PSNs accept risk. Two reactions emerged:

- State regulators allowed PSNs to assume risk from licensed health carriers without meeting HMO or insurer regulatory requirements. This frequently occurs in the form of capitation payments or other methods of risk-sharing between carriers and providers.

- Regulators are much less inclined to allow such unregulated risk assumption directly from employers.

Although the Balanced Budget Act of 1997 requires states to grant some regulatory flexibility to risk-assuming PSNs for Medicare managed care products, states are likely to continue to require such entities to meet regulatory requirements substantially similar to other risk-assuming health entities, such as HMOs and insurers.

Demands for Information

Justified or not, there is a widespread impression that consumers lack sufficient information about their health plans. Specifically, that missing information includes how to access care, how physicians are paid, and how to "work" the system. As a result, new legislation and regulations now require health plans to disclose more details about their operations to prospective buyers, members, and providers than they have in the past.

Why Information Is Important, and What Information Is Important

When consumers make choices about the goods and services they are buying, they must have some bases upon which to make those choices. In the case of health care, there are several kinds of choices, each driven by several criteria. In a system such as that which dominates the U.S. health financing market, employers choose the product, the design, and the supplier. Sometimes—more often in the case of small businesses—the choice ends there. With growing frequency, an employer gives the employee a choice of several products and suppliers that the employer initially selected. The size of the work force often dictates the number of choices provided by an employer: Larger organizations may offer multiple plans, while smaller employers frequently offer only one option.

What bases are employers and employees using to choose among the numerous health coverage options? As with most products and services, the criteria are usually reduced to either price or quality. However, unlike most products or services, the price of health coverage is substantial and the consequences of poor quality are profound.

The problem for health care consumers is that the information they need if they are to judge quality and price is dizzyingly complex:

■ Price is not just a single number, but a complex blend of up-front prices (in the form of premiums) and back-end costs (in the form of varying levels for deductibles, coinsurance, and copayments). Further, benefits often are not standardized, making price comparisons difficult or even meaningless.

■ Quality information is even more perplexing because of the differing perceptions about what constitutes quality care and quality service. For example, is "quality" suggested by the fact that a high percentage of the physicians on an MCO panel are board certified, or that the MCO has a short average waiting time on customer service calls? Is quality denoted by a health plan's having a high percentage of children who receive their immunizations before reaching the age of two, or a low number of member complaints? Each member's answer is likely to differ, depending on his or her personal situation.

What States and the NAIC Demand

Historically, states required carriers to disclose information that affected the price and design of the health coverage product. Rate regulation remains an important element of insurance regulation. New requirements in carrier disclosure insist on two things: (1) markers of health plan quality, and (2) uniformity of reporting methodology. The reason for these additions is clear: No longer is the information disclosed by carriers reviewed only by financial analysts and actuaries. New audiences—the consumers and purchasers of health coverage—influence the full-disclosure environment of the 1990s, one that is likely to persist into the next century. For these audiences, the data must be clear, comparable, and quality-focused.

Standardized reporting, as defined by the National Committee for Quality Assurance's (NCQA) *Health Plan Employer Data and Information Set* (HEDIS), provided a sound basis for comparable and interpretable reports on health plan quality indicators. States are building on this data set and others in their experiments with quality reporting formats. One example of the data that a state may require of health carriers and make available to the purchasing and consuming public is the Maryland Health Care Access and Cost Commission's HMO Quality Report Card. Available online and based in part on HEDIS data and in part on its own data requirements, this report examines a variety of measures of customer service, patient care, preventive health, and accreditation status.

Physician "Gag Clauses"

In 1995 and 1996, accusations abounded that managed care contracts with providers contained provisions that prohibited physicians from fully apprising their patients of their treatment options. These clauses also purportedly allowed health plans to stifle criticism by physicians. One professional medical association, for example, claimed that "Increasingly, HMOs and other health plans are incorporating 'gag' or 'confidentiality' clauses in their provider contracts, which expressly prohibit physicians from saying anything that could thwart the patient's confidence in the plan's policies and coverage."[28]

Legislatures responded with a flurry of activity. By the end of 1997, at least 40 states had adopted laws and/or regulations to limit or prohibit the use of "gag clauses" in provider contracts. Members of Congress also introduced legislation to prohibit these purported threats to the physician-patient relationship.[29] Interestingly, the U.S. General Accounting Office's examination of the issue found that, contrary to the widespread allegations of the medical community, gag clauses were virtually nonexistent in provider contracts.[30]

Good Housekeeping Seals: The Rise of Accreditation

As voters increasingly rely on regulators to ensure that health plans meet certain minimum quality standards, those regulators must search for markers of quality. While regulators strive to make their own assessments of health plan quality, lack of resources and expertise leads some states to depend on the approval of private accrediting institutions, such as NCQA, as one indicator of quality in health plans.

Although different accrediting organizations examine different aspects of a health plan's operations, all rely on rigorous audits of health plan operations to assess definitions of quality. The audits examine quality markers that range from clinical to operational to degree of customer satisfaction. These markers are precisely the sort of indicators that the public asks regulators to examine more closely. The question for these public overseers is whether to expand their teams of auditors to replicate activities of the private auditors, or to allow health plans to submit a passing grade from a designated organization as a substitute for some component—or even all—of government quality oversight.

Governments give credence to private accreditation of a health carrier in a variety of ways. Some states not only allow carriers to submit accreditation as a substitute for a state examination, but they also require it as one prerequisite of, or one of the requirements for, continuing business with the state.

■ Defining the Product

With the enactment of the Federal HMO Act of 1973, governments defined for managed care plans what they previously had defined for indemnity insurers:

the benefits that must be provided to consumers. As public confusion grows over the distinction between "medical necessity" as a boundary of health coverage and "medical necessity" as a clinical determination by the treating physician, so grow the attempts by public officials to define unilaterally "medical necessity," in the benefit-determination sense.

The History of State and Federal Definitions of the Product

Mandating specific benefits is not new to insurance or MCOs. Mandated benefits characterized insurance law for years. Even the seminal Federal HMO Act described Congress's notion of what benefits constituted the "comprehensive health coverage" required of all HMOs that qualified under the act. State HMO acts often blend existing insurance requirements with this federal notion of mandated benefits.

The number of benefits that health carriers are required to provide has expanded rapidly, with jurisdictions creating as few as two and as many as 45 mandated benefits. Historically, mandated benefits are descriptions of types of ailments to be treated or types of treatments to be provided. As MCOs and hospitals shorten hospital inpatient stays, however, these benefit mandates increasingly specify the duration of hospital stays for certain procedures.

Older mandates required coverage of certain procedures, such as mammograms or Pap smears, or the treatment of certain ailments, such as temporal mandibular joint syndrome (TMJ). Mandates that are more recent prescribe treatment modalities. For example, most states (and now Congress) prescribe minimum hospital lengths-of-stay for mothers and their newborn children, and many states adopted minimum lengths-of-stay for mastectomies.

Mental Health's Struggle for "Parity"

Historically, health carriers' restrictions on mental health coverage lacked counterparts in the domain of medical care. In response, behavioral health advocates campaigned to raise benefit levels for mental health services. The Mental Health Parity Act of 1996 (MHPA) requires that group plans that provide medical and mental health coverage not impose more restrictive annual and lifetime dollar limits on mental health benefits than they do on medical benefits.

To advocates of mental health "parity," the MHPA is only a partial victory because it does not prevent health carriers from otherwise placing limits on the duration, amount, or scope of mental health benefits. In 1997, 12 states enacted mental health mandates, and many others are likely to follow. Bills under consideration at the state and national level require health carriers to provide mental health benefits that are more generous. Advocates typically push for legislation that requires the terms and conditions of coverage for mental health conditions to be at least as generous as those for physical illness. Some proposals require that deductibles, copayments, and number of covered inpatient days and/or outpatient visits match those for medical coverage. These more aggressive bills face stiff opposition from employers concerned about the affordability of mandated mental health coverage.

The Mandated Benefits Process

Payer, purchaser, and provider organizations see the rush toward increases in mandated benefits as a threat both to plan solvency and to physician dominance of clinical decisions. There also appears to be a realization that the state and federal legislatures are poor arenas for these types of operational decisions. In response, organizations advocate mechanisms for more rational evaluations, both clinical and economic, of proposed new mandates. Some states (such as Virginia) use a process by which a commission, outside the normal legislative process, evaluates proposed mandates for clinical efficacy and economic impact. A growing number of states are considering similar mechanisms as a brake on the burgeoning number—and cost—of mandated benefits.

Maryland's approach to limiting mandated benefits in its small group market is gaining credibility. In that state, an independent commission (not the legislature) decides which state mandates applicable to the large group commercial market should apply to the small group market (up to a certain dollar limit that is tied to the average annual wage in the state). Should the cost of the comprehensive benefit plan exceed that limit, the commission must decide which benefits to remove to lower the total cost of mandated benefits under the ceiling established by the law.

■ Provider Networks

A central feature of managed care is the use of provider networks. Not surprisingly, provider networks are often targets for criticism and, increasingly, new regulatory schemes, especially if the network receives a capitated payment. Providers complained about health plans' limiting their access to the networks, and consumers objected to limited access to providers that do not participate in such panels. Finally, some health plans' operations of the networks engendered both complaints and regulation.

Provider Membership in the Network

In all provider networks, no matter the model, the central fact is this: Some providers in the community will be in, and some will be out. This is especially true of physicians. In a given area, however, there usually is a sufficient number of physicians to exclude many and still satisfy consumers. In the early days of managed care, when HMO market share was small, it was the HMOs—hat in hand—that sought physicians to join the nascent organizations. Now, in those areas of the country where a much greater percentage of the insured population relies on MCOs, it is the physicians who are seeking—again, hat in hand— to join the very panels they shunned only a few years ago.

One legal approach, advocated by providers and provider organizations seeking to gain access to restricted provider panels, is the "any willing provider" law (AWP). Under an AWP law, a payer that operates through a network of providers is required to accept into that panel any appropriately licensed provider that agrees to the terms of participation required of the other providers on the panel. MCOs argue that an AWP law erodes their ability to manage the quality of the panel and negotiate discounts with providers. In turn, providers argue that it is fundamentally unfair to allow MCOs to choose among providers to form a panel. Some courts found that ERISA preempts AWP laws because eliminating limited provider networks directly affects the structure, content, and administration of health benefit plans (i.e., the business of insurance).[31]

Member Access Outside the Network

Another policy debate surrounding provider networks involves the member's ability to obtain covered benefits from providers who are not participating in a plan's network. The most common public approach to this issue is the "mandatory point-of-service" law. A point-of-service (POS) product allows the member coverage for care obtained from providers outside of the provider network, usually at some additional cost (in terms of more limited benefits). Under a mandatory POS law, plans are required to offer at least the employer (and in some states, the employee) a choice between a closed-panel HMO and either a POS product or an indemnity insurance product (e.g., a preferred provider organization [PPO]).

Advocates of POSs ran into legal difficulties in their efforts to gain mandates for this option. Courts and attorneys generally agree that, while a state may mandate that an insurer offer the employer an option to buy a POS or indemnity product, ERISA prohibits a mandate that the offer extend to the employee. This emerging case law has not prevented some states from adopting mandatory

POS laws that extend the offer to the employee, but the most common approach limits the offer to the employer.[32]

Direct Access to Specialists

"Direct access" laws allow HMO members to bypass health plan requirements that they obtain referrals to covered specialty services from a primary care provider (PCP). These laws respond to yet another criticism of the MCO network. Typically, MCOs coordinate care and review utilization by channeling access to medical specialists through PCPs. Some states attack this practice either through "direct access" laws for certain specialties or by allowing members to select certain medical specialists as their PCPs. Obstetrics and gynecology, dermatology, chiropractic, and nurse practitioners are specialties included in state direct access statutes.

■ Regulating the Payer-Provider Relationship

MCOs operate primarily through a provider contract mechanism. The relationship defined by the contract determines the risk-sharing and apportionment of money between payer and provider, the quality mandates, and the sanction mechanisms. It is no surprise that the relationship between payer and provider is the focus of growing regulatory interest.

Capitation, Withholds, and Bonuses

Many MCOs compensate at least some of the providers in their panels through "capitation." Most capitation arrangements tie PCP compensation to the number of plan members who select the provider as their PCP. A capitated arrangement for a specialist often ties compensation to an estimate of the portion of the MCO's members served by that specialist.

The policy concern that surrounds capitated provider arrangements arises from a perception that such arrangements prompt the provider to withhold medically necessary care. MCOs counter-argue that capitated arrangements only affect overutilization, not proper utilization, and that the requirements of professional practice and the fear of malpractice liability sufficiently deter physicians from providing less care than is medically necessary.

Despite the critics of capitation, such agreements are increasingly popular. Nearly 60 percent of physician groups report receiving some compensation under capitation arrangements; another 30 percent expect the same by 2000.[33] One study published in the *New England Journal of Medicine* concluded that, while the "jury was still out" on the quality concerns raised by capitation's critics, "It can be said with certainty that the empirical literature as a whole so far does not make capitation out to be the villain that some believe it is."[34]

Capitation is not the only financial incentive available to health carriers. Some MCOs establish withhold and bonus systems as incentives to participating providers. A "withhold" typically is a portion of an MCO's payment to a provider that is withheld during a time period, and the payment of the amount withheld is contingent upon the fulfillment by the provider of certain conditions tied to quality, administrative, or utilization issues. A bonus—the other side of the withhold—is a payment beyond the base arrangement that monetarily rewards certain behavior sought by the MCO.

Despite the lack of clear evidence that capitation arrangements or bonus compensation methodologies pose quality-of-care problems, states are examining ways to regulate their use. The variety of proposed methods include:

- requiring capitation rates to be actuarially sound;[35]

- requiring that financial incentives or provider payment mechanisms be disclosed to MCO members;[36] and

- prohibiting incentives or "payment made directly, in any form, to a health care provider or health care provider group as an inducement to deny, reduce, limit, or delay specific, medically necessary, and appropriate services provided with respect to a specific insured or groups of insureds with similar medical conditions."[37]

Physician Incentive Plans: The New Federal Regulations

The federal government has yet to express concern about modest financial incentives for providers, but it did enter the fray with laws and impending regulations to limit incentives when the provider is placed at substantial financial risk. In 1996, the Health Care Financing Administration promulgated Physician Incentive Plan Regulations implementing amendments to the Social Security Act enacted in the Comprehensive Omnibus Budget Reconciliation Act of 1993.[38] These regulations are a complicated attempt to limit the extent to which a provider may assume substantial financial risk as related to the amount or type of care delivered. The regulations generally define "substantial financial risk" as occurring when "the incentive arrangements place the physician or physician group at-risk for amounts beyond [25 percent], if the risk is based on the use or costs of referral services."

Payment for Emergency Services

Federal law and MCO practices are stimulating substantial discussion among the states regarding the payment of emergency room physicians and hospitals that operate emergency rooms. The Emergency Medical Treatment and Active Labor Act (EMTALA) requires any hospital with an emergency department to conduct an appropriate medical screening examination on all individuals who seek care to determine whether or not they are experiencing an emergency medical condition.[39] If it is determined that an emergency medical condition exists, the hospital must stabilize the patient's condition or transfer the patient to another facility if stabilization is not possible. A hospital may not delay the screening examination to inquire about an individual's method of payment or insurance status.

MCOs cover emergency care but discourage members from using emergency rooms for non-emergency medical care. That position gives rise to disputes between MCOs and emergency physicians and hospitals about payment when an MCO member seeks treatment for a non-emergency condition in an emergency facility. Hospitals and emergency physicians argue that because federal law requires that they screen and stabilize all patients (even those appearing not to have an emergency condition) the MCO should pay for at least the screening and stabilizing treatment. MCOs argue that forcing them to pay for treatment of non-emergency conditions in emergency facilities removes the financial incentives the MCOs need to encourage members to use settings that are more appropriate for non-emergency care.

States and the federal government respond to these public policy arguments in several ways:

- Redefining "emergency" in an effort to clarify the circumstances under which MCOs must pay for treatment in an emergency facility. Most states that take this approach opt for a subjective definition (commonly called the "reasonable or prudent layperson standard") that focuses on whether a reasonable person, with a layperson's understanding of medicine, would believe that immediate care was needed.

- Requiring such features as 24-hour access to health care professionals to help determine whether there is a medical emergency.

- Requiring payment for screening, stabilization, and maintenance of care in non-emergency and emergency cases.

Drugs: Formularies and Other Pharmacy Issues

Health carriers attempt to contain rising pharmaceutical costs in several ways. The most prevalent method is the adoption of "formularies," which MCOs use as incentives for members and physicians to select the lower-cost alternatives when there are choices among clinically equivalent prescription drugs. These formularies seldom come into play when the prescribing physician explicitly indicates that a particular drug must be "dispensed as written." The controversy occurs when the physician, by remaining silent on the issue, allows substitutions of clinically equivalent alternatives listed on a formulary.

Opponents of formularies attack their use by proposing a variety of restrictions. In 1997, seven states adopted laws affecting the use of formularies, and more states are likely to consider similar mandates. Anti-formulary laws take several forms; they may:

- simply require the use of open formularies (penalizes, but does not prohibit, the use of drugs not on the formulary);

- prohibit the use of formularies altogether; or

- specify minimum disclosure requirements regarding the use of formularies.

Another group of proposed laws establishes procedures to cover non-formulary drugs.

■ Utilization Review and Appeals and Grievances

Despite existing laws that govern the processes by which members and providers may appeal the decisions of MCOs, both groups complain about the unresponsiveness or incomprehensibility of such processes in some health plans. These complaints led policy makers to develop new systems of oversight for processing appeals and grievances.

Existing Requirements

Health plans are accountable for coverage decisions under both public law and the private accreditation process. The laws include the Federal HMO Act, federal laws and regulations concerning Medicare and Medicaid, state insurance laws, and state HMO laws. Additionally, private accreditation agencies, such as NCQA, the American Accreditation Healthcare Commission, and the Utilization Review Accreditation Commission (URAC), impose rigorous requirements for appeals and grievances on plans that seek accreditation. Such requirements generally cover the qualifications of those who make coverage decisions, due process requirements, and time limits for responses to appeals.

Demands for Clarity, Access, and Accountability

Despite the plethora of existing requirements concerning the review of coverage decisions, some states adopted (or are considering) laws that strengthen health plan accountability. The more moderate proposals require improvement in the mechanisms MCOs use to review coverage decisions. The more radical approach (one that is the subject of vehement debate in policy circles) expands existing tort liability to include liability for injuries proximately caused by carelessly made coverage decisions.

Improving Appeals and Grievance Systems

Much of the recent activity over accountability for coverage decisions takes the form of legislation that requires mechanisms, external to the health plan, to review those decisions. Such bills usually require a member to exhaust a plan's internal procedures for appealing coverage decisions, and then allows for appeal to an external agency. Some states allow the member to make that appeal to an entity established by the state, while others allow the plans to designate the external appeal agents.[40] Some of these bills establish mechanisms to expedite review of coverage decisions.[41]

Tort Liability

As the tort liability of physicians was a controversial issue in the 1970s and 1980s, the tort liability of MCOs and their medical directors is the hot issue of the late 1990s. Although ERISA and the Federal HMO Act provide some liability protection for MCOs, that protection is neither comprehensive nor permanent.

Potential tort liability for MCOs. Under ERISA, an MCO's liability for incorrect coverage decisions is limited to the value of the benefit denied. That limitation prohibits MCO members from suing in tort to recover from an ERISA "plan" for injuries suffered as a result of an MCO's wrongful denial of a benefit.

Another principle of law—*respondeat superior*—provides for MCO liability for injuries caused by the breach of duty of ordinary care by the treating provider but only when that provider is an employee of the MCO. Because most Americans are covered by MCOs that contract with private physicians on an independent contractor basis, however, members often cannot bring actions against their MCO in tort if they suffer injury through the negligence of their treating providers.

Broadening tort law. In 1997, a health plan liability issue that attracted national attention was Texas Governor George Bush, Jr.'s decision to decline to veto a bill (SB 386) to create a new cause of action against health plans. This law provides that health carriers owe a duty of ordinary care when making treatment decisions and that breach of the duty exposes carriers to liability for "damages for harm to an insured or enrollee proximately caused by its failure to exercise ordinary care."

The potential reach of this law is substantial. Under the law, health carriers are "liable for damages for harm to an insured or an enrollee proximately caused by the health care treatment decisions made by its employees; agents; ostensible agents; or representatives who are acting on its behalf and over whom it has the right to exercise influence or control, or has actually exercised influence or control." Plaintiffs are expected to argue that, given the nature of financial arrangements between carriers and providers, they "are acting on [the carriers'] behalf," exposing the carrier to liability to which it was previously not exposed.

There is a question about the legality, under ERISA, of this law. In pending litigation that challenges the Texas statute, carriers argue that state law can have no impact on the federal preemption embodied in ERISA. Despite the uncertainty about the legality of this law, several dozen bills are under consideration by legislatures across the country that affect health plan liability.

State Licensure Issues Regarding Medical Directors and Nurses

Another issue related to health plan liability concerns the question of whether utilization review constitutes the practice of medicine. The health carriers' position is that utilization review is simply a benefit determination, even when it involves the question of "medical necessity." They argue that none of the normal indications of a physician-patient relationship (such as face-to-face contact) exists and that "necessity," as determined in connection with a coverage question, differs from a judgment of medical necessity rendered by a treating physician. Critics counter with the argument that the practical effect of a denial of coverage is, for many patients, the denial of care itself and, therefore, is *de facto* identical to the practice of medicine.

Some state boards of medicine (agencies that license medical professionals to practice in a state) are beginning to insist that they have authority over medical directors and nurses performing utilization review functions. At least two dozen states have considered and rejected bills to establish boards of medical authority over utilization review and to hold medical directors responsible for treatment policies, protocols, quality assurance activities, and utilization management decisions of the MCO.

◼ Conclusion

In the late 1990s and the next decade, the regulation of health plans is certain to change substantially, for several reasons:

■ First, regulation, of necessity, follows changes in the marketplace. Because the health financing market is destined to undergo radical changes in the next decade and beyond, regulators need new tools and approaches just to maintain their present level of oversight.

■ Second, health care regulation is increasingly a federal, not just a state, issue. The mid- to late-1990s produced the first substantial federal health initiatives beyond the domains of Medicare, Medicaid, and Social Security. These initiatives piqued the interest of members of Congress, interest groups, and consumers regarding a heretofore little-used vehicle for insurance regulation: the federal government. This interest is almost sure to grow, and the battle for hegemony between the states and the federal government is likely to keep everyone who is involved in health policy busy for years to come.

■ Third, regulatory and market forces will continue to push against each other to create substantial political dynamism.

These pressures toward increased regulation will continue to collide with equally powerful pressures to limit the costs associated with that regulation. Every heartfelt plea for a regulatory requirement will be met with an equally sincere plea to reduce costs, to give more Americans access to affordable health coverage. Every effort to create greater accountability by health plans will collide with equivalent efforts to decrease providers' accountability to health plans. Americans want it both ways: unlimited services at a limited cost. It is likely to be a very long time before the health care policy discussion becomes sufficiently mature to acknowledge that every benefit has its price. Until then, there will be much wheel-spinning in the halls of legislatures and bureaucracies to sort out those benefits and regulations that Americans are willing to pay for from those they are not.

■ Key Terms

Accreditation

Appeals and grievance systems

the "business of insurance"

Capitation

"Confidentiality" clauses

Consolidated Licensure for Entities Assuming Risk (CLEAR)

Emergency Medical Treatment and Active Labor Act (EMTALA)

ERISA preemption

Federal HMO Act

Limits of state regulatory authority

Mandated benefits

Maryland Health Care Access and Cost Commission's HMO Quality Report Card

Mental health parity

National Association of Insurance Commissioners (NAIC)

NCQA'S *Health Plan Employer Data and Information Set* (HEDIS)

Payer and medical director liability

Provider networks

Provider-sponsored network (PSN)

Risk-bearing entities

Utilization review

Utilization Review Accreditation Commission (URAC)

Vertical/horizontal industry regulation

Virginia Bureau of Insurance (VBOI)

Chapter 3

MANAGED CARE AND THE CONSUMER

■ Introduction

In the first half of the 20th century, medical societies branded managed care organizations (known then as prepaid group practice plans) as socialist entities that attracted inferior doctors and provided an inferior quality of care. Managed care organizations represented such a small part of the health care delivery system that they lacked market power and were largely ignored.

By the end of the 1980s, health care costs accounted for 12 percent of the U.S. gross domestic product (GDP), in contrast to approximately 7 percent of the GDPs of Japan and most European countries. Despite the extra health care spending, however, life expectancy in the United States lagged behind that in both Europe and Japan.[42] A popular belief emerged that health care costs no longer reflected economic reality, a view reinforced by major newspapers and magazines that published extensive articles about health care costs in the United States. In the early 1990s, managed care became the dominant solution for employers and consumers to help lower cost and improve quality.

During the past few years, the managed care industry has found itself frequently in a defensive posture. Many of the cost control virtues touted in the late 1980s and early 1990s are now seen in a negative light. MCOs' support for limiting care to appropriate procedures only and for reduced hospital lengths-of-stay are now perceived as denying consumers necessary care to increase corporate profits. Many physicians, hospital personnel, and other care providers resent the imposition of MCOs in their operations and the impact on their revenue streams, but they acknowledge that managed care does force the system to be more efficient. MCOs successfully reined in double-digit health inflation, but at the expense of relationships with providers. Strained relationships with providers contributed to the consumer backlash against managed care, resulting in new regulations and legislation that force MCOs to change their business strategies.

Consumers React to Managed Care

Today MCOs, as a dominant force in the health care delivery system, are no longer ignored. Early 1990s polling data consistently showed that consumers were satisfied with the care they received from MCOs. During the 1994 health care reform debate, surveys revealed that the public did not believe that the government could solve the cost problems in health care, and wanted the market to do so. This perception led, in large part, to the defeat of President Clinton's health care reform effort.

In the mid-1990s, as consumers' choices regarding their health care services decreased, there was a growing negative perception of managed care. This perception was revealed in polling data:

- A 1995 survey sponsored by the Commonwealth Fund Foundation found that 21 percent of managed care enrollees rated their plan as fair or poor, compared with 14 percent of fee-for-service users. The survey also found that managed care enrollees were less satisfied than fee-for-service enrollees in the areas of doctor choice, changing physicians, and the quality of health care providers.[43]

- In the two years from 1995 to 1997, consumer perceptions of managed care continued to decline. In a 1997 Kaiser Family Foundation survey, 33 percent of fee-for-service enrollees gave their plan an "A" rating, while only 22 percent of managed care enrollees rated their plan that high. In the same survey, 32 percent of managed care enrollees gave their plan a rating of "C" or below compared with 19 percent of fee-for-service enrollees. The survey also found that:

  - 36 percent of HMOs did a good job.

  - 34 percent of managed care companies did a good job.

  - 61 percent of the public believed that managed care decreased the time doctors spend with patients.

  - 59 percent of the public believed that managed care made it harder for the sick to see medical specialists.

- 55 percent believed that managed care had not made much difference in reducing health care costs.
- 51 percent believed that managed care had decreased the quality of care to the sick.[44]

Poll data show a continuing decrease in consumer confidence in the medical system. This is most pronounced in the public's view toward for-profit health care organizations. For a number of years, the Kaiser Family Foundation Surveys asked consumers whether a for-profit or not-for-profit health plan provides better quality care. A March 1997 survey found that 48 percent of the public felt that a for-profit health plan would provide better quality care, while 38 percent said that a not-for-profit plan would. By January 1998, the same question elicited a different response: 30 percent stated that a for-profit health plan would be the better provider of quality care, while 46 percent voted for a not-for-profit plan.[45] This is a remarkable turnaround in only nine months and reflects the growing unhappiness among consumers with the U.S. health care system.

The January 1998 poll also found that 72 percent of Americans favor a consumer bill of rights, similar to the one proposed in 1997 by the President's Advisory Commission on Consumer Protection and Quality in the Health Care Industry.[46] However, the support level for such a bill drops from 74 percent to 43 percent if it increases consumers' insurance premiums by $1 to $5 per month and drops to 28 percent for a $15 to $20 per month increase. Additionally, the poll found that 65 percent of consumers oppose additional managed care regulation if it resulted in a small number of employers dropping health care coverage. This number grows to 73 percent if additional regulation resulted in a large number of employers dropping health care coverage.

The poll also shows that consumers are far less concerned with government involvement in health care than they were four years ago.

- By a 48 to 38 percent margin, consumers support "somewhat more" government involvement in health care.
- A plurality of 45 percent support a "lot more" government involvement in health care.
- 57 percent believe that regulation of the managed care industry should be performed by a nongovernmental entity.

The 1998 Health Confidence Survey showed that, while people favor additional consumer protections, most people in managed care plans are satisfied with the care they currently receive. The survey found the following:

- 52 percent of consumers are satisfied with their health plans and 36 percent are somewhat satisfied.

- 61 percent rate the quality of care in managed care plans as better than that of other insurance options.
- 47 percent say managed care gives consumers a choice of hospitals.
- 46 percent say managed care gives consumers a choice of doctors.
- 46 percent say managed care gives consumers access to specialists.
- 42 percent say managed care gives consumers access to preventive care.

Much of the polling data support the popular public opinion that the current managed care system is too restrictive and is starting to lower quality of care overall. However, the public remains very concerned about the continued increases in their health care costs. They want a consumer bill of rights, but they don't want large increases in health insurance premiums.

The Press and Politics

Since the mid-1990s, media coverage of managed care has been increasingly negative. It is always difficult to determine whether the media drives or reflects public opinion. However, media recognition of the public's concern about the quality of managed care is clear. All three major network news programs, plus CNN, *Time, Newsweek, U.S. News & World Report*, and most of the major daily newspapers, produced extensive articles detailing anecdotal problems that they termed "managed care abuses."

The issue of consumer concern with managed care has also reached into popular culture. In the movie *As Good As It Gets*, the heroine curses her HMO's failure to properly treat her son's asthma. Her statement elicits one of the audience's most positive vocal reactions.

Media attention contributes to legislation and to regulation of the industry. For example:

- A *Time* magazine cover in 1996 featured a doctor with a gag over his mouth, to illustrate a feature article relating how managed care doctors are restricted from telling patients about all available treatment by the so-called gag clauses in doctor contracts. This type of coverage contributed to the "anti-gag" language contained in the 1997 Medicare program legislation and in bills passed by many state legislatures.
- Media stories about denial of services by health plans also affect the industry. The most celebrated example involved Nelene Fox, whose story was covered by *Time* and many network news programs. Ms. Fox suffered from an advanced form of breast cancer and sought a bone marrow transplant as a possible cure. The procedure was considered experimental by her insurer

(Health Net), which denied coverage. Ms. Fox eventually died from breast cancer; her family sued Health Net and won an $89 million judgment. Subsequently, Health Net decided to settle the suit rather than appeal.

As a result of the publicity surrounding the Fox case, many state legislatures mandated health plans to cover autologous bone marrow transplants for the treatment of advanced breast cancer. In late 1994, the Federal Employees Health Benefits Program included autologous bone marrow transplants in its benefits package, despite inconclusive evidence as to whether the procedure was experimental.

In early 1997, the media reported on MCOs that performed some mastectomies on an outpatient basis. The public outcry produced by these stories resulted in the introduction of a number of bills in Congress that require a minimum length-of-stay of 48 hours for a mastectomy. This occurred even though only a limited number of mastectomies were performed on an outpatient basis.

The media, which once offered only occasional commentaries on managed care, came to act as one its most prominent detractors. As the focus of public concern moved from the high cost of health care to the quality of care, the media followed suit. Stories today generally credit managed care for enforcing some discipline in the health care system, but question whether the emphasis on cost control affects quality. If the public's opinion of managed care continues to erode, the media is likely to continue its negative coverage.

■ Politicians and Consumer Protection

Managed care in the early 1990s became the preferred vehicle to contain health cost inflation and played a central part in President Clinton's 1994 health care reform proposal. Despite managed care's growing market share, MCOs, small businesses, and doctors disliked many aspects of the Clinton plan and lobbied, successfully, for its defeat.

Politicians watch the polls closer than anyone, and the current consumer protection laws are traceable to the public's perceptions about managed care. While legislation that called for increasing regulations once rested squarely in the Democrats' domain, the unhappiness with managed care prompted normally business-friendly Republicans to support increased government oversight of health plans. Some examples:

■ In 1995, New Jersey (a state with a Republican governor and state legislature) enacted the first 48-hour maternity length-of-stay bill and passed some of the toughest managed care consumer protection laws in the country.

41

■ The two most vocal critics of managed care in Congress, Representatives Greg Ganske (Iowa) and Charlie Norwood (Georgia), are both conservative Republicans. Congressman Norwood introduced a tough managed care consumer protection bill, currently pending in Congress, with more than 200 co-sponsors, almost half Republicans.

It is likely that state and federal policy makers will continue to respond to consumer issues and that many piecemeal bills will be introduced to increase consumer protections in health care plans.

■ Consumer Issues

Consumer Access to Information

Widespread access to new information sources (such as the Internet) increases consumers' knowledge about every product they purchase, including health care. Consumers expect to be able to obtain information about their health care providers, treatment coverage options, quality of care, and costs, and they express frustration when that information is not available to them. This frustration is evident in a recent survey that found 92 percent of Americans favored a law requiring health plans to provide information about plan operations, covered benefits, participating doctors, and procedures to resolve grievances.

This demand for information is met in a variety of ways by both the private and public sectors. For example, a number of states enacted comprehensive managed care consumer protection laws, with requirements that health care plans disclose, for example, covered services, cost-sharing requirements, physician information (including credentials), utilization review procedures, emergency and out-of-area coverage, and grievance and appeals mechanisms.

In addition, several independent organizations measure health care and the results are reported for consumer use:

■ The National Committee for Quality Assurance (NCQA)
NCQA's HEDIS data are so widely known and respected that *U.S. News & World Report* used HEDIS measurements in its late-1997 report ranking HMOs by quality. Many corporations use HEDIS ratings to determine the quality of care provided by HMOs, and some require NCQA accreditation for participation. Additionally, Medicare requires its HMO contractors to provide yearly HEDIS measurements on its members, and many states require health plans to report Medicaid HEDIS data as well.

■ Foundation for Accountability (FACCT)
Founded in 1995, FACCT focuses on health outcomes. It examines health

plans by assessing how well they keep members healthy, how well they help enrollees recover from illness or live with chronic illness, and how an MCO adapts to the changing needs of its members. In late 1997, FACCT published its results on 100 of the nation's largest HMOs. *Newsweek* used the FACCT survey results in a December 15, 1997 article to advise people on how to choose a health plan.

■ The Agency for Health Care Policy and Research (AHCPR)
AHCPR (a federal program in the U.S. Department of Health and Human Services) developed the Consumer Assessment of Health Plans Survey (CAHPS), a standard survey to measure both health plan quality and consumer satisfaction. The CAHPS survey has become the standard consumer survey instrument for the industry. NCQA has incorporated CAHPS into its Member Satisfaction Survey and plans to include it in its 1999 HEDIS reporting requirements.

The "information highway" has rapidly transported us to an era in which a great deal of information is accessible to many people. This additional information is necessary and helpful to consumers, but it can also create confusion, such as when report cards from NCQA and FACCT show different results for the same health plan. As more organizations rank managed care plans, it is possible that consumers will demand one set of standards that will allow them to compare health plans based on quality of care and services.

Consumer Information and Privacy

Modern technology raises concerns about people's privacy in a number of areas, including health care. In the paper age, individuals felt that their medical records were secure in a locked file cabinet in their doctor's office. Now, a great deal of medical information is on computers, making access to it easier for both authorized and unauthorized personnel. While these electronic records are generally as secure as they would be in a locked file cabinet (in some cases, more secure), public concern has been heightened by a series of highly publicized incidents in which medical records have been released to the press.

In an effort to address this issue, the Clinton administration developed medical record confidentiality standards that protect the consumer but also permit needed medical research and quality assurance programs to continue. In September 1997, the administration issued its report on medical records confidentiality and recommended:

1. Establishing the patient as the owner of medical records, with health plans, hospitals, and doctors as custodians.

43

2. Defining specific rules for the use of medical records without patient authorization, including payment of health care services, medical research, public health purposes, quality assurance activities, accreditation and licensure, and fraud and abuse prevention. In almost all other cases, the patient's permission is needed to view his or her medical record.

3. Allowing patients to request copies of their medical records and make corrections.

4. Requiring the custodian of the medical record to document each instance in which the record is accessed.

Congress received these recommendations, but, by mid-1998, had yet to act on them. Several members of Congress are also working on their own proposals for medical records confidentiality. Senator Robert Bennett (R-Utah), a leader in this area, has twice introduced the Medical Records Privacy Act in Congress. This bill is restrictive and permits only limited use of medical records for purposes such as payment of health care bills. In almost all other cases, the patient's authorization would be necessary to access a medical record. Senator Bennett realizes that his bill is too restrictive and is working to address concerns about the impact of these restrictions on medical research and quality assurance programs.

Consumer Choice

Managed care generally produces lower costs and more efficient medical services, but often reduces consumers' choice of providers. Employers often limit the number of health plan options as a means to obtain better prices. Large businesses, along with state and federal governments, provide multiple health coverage options, but many small businesses offer only one plan. In a 1995 Commonwealth Foundation Survey, 30 percent of managed care members reported no fee-for-service option.

More health plans are responding to consumer issues about choice limitations by expanding the networks of physicians available to their members. Additionally, more employers request a point-of-service (POS) option. POS plans are popular because they give managed care enrollees the security of knowing they can seek care outside the network, if they choose.

In addition to the market movement toward greater choice, some states mandate that health plans provide a POS option to their enrollees. New York requires that all MCOs provide a POS option in their individual markets, and New Jersey requires that all plans operating in the state offer a POS option. A number of consumer protection bills, pending on both the state and federal level, mandate a POS option. As managed care continues to be the dominant health care delivery method, the debate over choice of health plan or provider is likely to continue.

▉ Instituting Consumer Protection Standards

Polling data demonstrate the public belief that MCOs need more oversight from an entity outside the industry. A recent poll shows that:

- 34 percent of the public want managed care regulated by an independent entity.
- 19 percent want managed care regulated by the federal government.
- 18 percent want managed care regulated by the state governments.
- 16 percent don't want managed care regulated at all.

In response, competing initiatives and a variety of consumer regulation laws are emerging from the federal and state governments.

Industry Initiatives

The managed care industry hopes to avoid government regulation through voluntary, industry-sponsored programs. The Health Insurance Association of America (HIAA), American Association of Health Plans (AAHP), American Hospital Association, and others argue that many health plans already perform the functions mandated in consumer protection legislation and that government regulation stifles innovation in health care delivery and quality assurance.

Beyond the accreditation and quality reporting mechanisms mentioned above, HIAA and other industry groups have set standards or guidelines focused on consumer rights and protections that are designed to build consumer confidence in managed care.

Despite industry efforts to better inform consumers, polling data from a variety of sources (ranging from the Kaiser Family Foundation to Republican pollster Frank Luntz) show that consumers are not happy with the fact that they have to rely on newspapers or employers for information on physicians and health plans. History demonstrates that Congress and state legislatures tend to step in when they believe that the public needs protection. Given today's environment, it remains to be seen whether the managed care industry convinces Congress to permit self-regulation.

State Initiatives

Already experienced in regulating health plans, the states took the lead in establishing consumer protection mechanisms. In recent years, several states have passed, and others are considering, sweeping managed care reforms to provide comprehensive consumer protections.

New York

In spring 1996, New York passed a comprehensive consumer protection bill for managed care enrollees. The law increases health plan accountability and improves the information available to consumers. The law requires plans operating in New York to:

1. ensure that the network has a sufficient number of physicians to serve its population;
2. permit chronically ill patients to select a specialist as their primary care physician;
3. disclose detailed information regarding coverage, utilization review, and physician selection criteria;
4. pay for emergency services based on the "prudent layperson" concept;
5. establish an internal appeals procedure for patients who are denied care;
6. establish due process rights for physicians facing termination; and
7. eliminate "gag" clauses from all provider contracts.

New Jersey

Like New York, New Jersey adopted an "HMO Consumer Bill of Rights" for managed care enrollees in 1996. The rules are the result of a two-year process involving a 32-member task force composed of health plan representatives, physicians, nurses, hospital associations, businesses, and consumers. The New Jersey regulations require health plans to:

1. ensure that the network has a sufficient number of physicians to serve its population;
2. permit chronically ill patients to select a specialist as their primary care physician;
3. disclose detailed information regarding coverage, utilization review, and physician selection criteria;
4. establish due process rights for physicians facing termination; and
5. eliminate "gag" clauses from all provider contracts.

Unlike New York, New Jersey established a non-binding external review board for patients who exhaust the internal grievance procedure. While decisions of the external review board are non-binding, large fines are imposed if the state finds that an MCO is not abiding by the board's decisions, thus effectively negating the non-binding attribute.

California

California, traditionally a bellwether state for national trends, foreshadows the future for the managed care industry. In 1997, the California legislature passed more than 90 bills that increased state regulation of MCOs. Governor Pete Wilson vetoed most of the bills, while awaiting a report from his 30-member commission on managed care. The commission, charged with developing recommendations for managed care quality, access, and cost, released its report in January 1998. It recommended the following:

1. Creating a new state entity to regulate HMOs, medical groups, and other provider organizations that bear significant risk. PPOs and fee-for-service plans would fall under the responsibility of this agency within two years.
2. Establishing risk adjusters in most insurance markets.
3. Establishing utilization management procedures that incorporate pre-credentialing, practice guidelines, clinical pathways, and outcomes data.
4. Establishing an independent third-party review process to address grievances and appeals.
5. Prohibiting capitation of individual physicians for a substantial portion of the cost of referrals.
6. Permitting pregnant women and patients treated for chronic illness who involuntarily change plans to continue treatment with their current provider for up to 90 days, or until the patient "safely transitions" to a new provider.
7. Developing five standard "reference contracts" for HMO, PPO, POS, and indemnity products.
8. Offering consumers a choice of health plans, whenever possible.
9. Involving consumers in the governing body and member advisory committees of MCOs.
10. Encouraging health plans to move toward credentialing and certifying medical groups and providers based on their knowledge, sensitivity, skills, and cultural competence to serve vulnerable populations.[47]

These recommendations far surpass the New York and New Jersey statutes. They are under consideration by the governor and the state legislature, and even more far-reaching reforms are possible.

Texas

Texas has followed the trend of providing more extensive consumer information to managed care plan members. In 1997, Dan Morales, the state attorney general, prohibited the state insurance department from disclosing the information contained in complaints against health plans. However, in May 1998, the attorney general reversed his ruling, stating that most complaints filed with the insurance department are now public. The public can know about complaints filed against HMOs. Health plans are concerned that the ruling will result in the release of confidential information, such as patient medical records or contract agreements with providers. The Texas decision could lead more states to disclose coverage denials and other complaints against health plans.

NAIC Model Acts

In addition to the actions of individual states, the National Association of Insurance Commissioners (NAIC) developed guidelines for states to use to establish managed care consumer protection laws. The model acts cover the areas of access to services, quality assurance programs, medical record confidentiality, disclosure of information to consumers, emergency care, non-discrimination against providers and beneficiaries, and provider credentialing. Many states use NAIC model acts to develop their health insurance laws and regulations. The use of the NAIC guidelines signals an interest by states to apply consumer protection standards to MCOs.

Federal Initiatives

With a sense of the issue's political potency, both Republicans and Democrats in Congress are scrambling to claim the political high ground in this debate. House and Senate Democrats have introduced expansive legislation that would establish a consumer's right to sue his or her health plan for medical malpractice, create an external appeals process, provide access to care standards, require a mandatory POS option, and set minimum information disclosure standards. House and Senate Republican task forces are working to produce a narrower bill that intrudes less on the operations of health plans.

Federal consumer protection regulation for managed care has advantages and disadvantages. Regulations can be advantageous if they preempt state laws to create one national standard. Such a standard would provide the consumer with uniform protection across the country and would give MCOs unified compliance systems, a single disclosure document, a single data-reporting system, and further consolidation of consumer protection activities. Those changes would be especially helpful to MCOs that operate in multiple states.

What are the disadvantages of regulation? The federal government does have experience in regulating companies participating in the Medicare and Medicaid programs, but lacks experience in regulating commercial health insurance. It also lacks the bureaucratic infrastructure to support this type of regulatory activity. The lack of understanding of the industry and its institutional knowledge is likely to create confusion in the regulatory process. Further, increased regulation and mandatory requirements generally contribute to higher costs for health care coverage.

Health Insurance Portability and Accountability Act (HIPAA)

The 1996 passage of HIPAA puts the federal government in the business of regulating health insurance. This complex law sets basic federal guidelines for pre-existing conditions and renewability of large and small group health insurance. Under HIPAA, states are required to adjust their health insurance laws to comply with the new federal law. If a state fails to make the necessary changes, the federal government assumes the governing function for those areas covered by the law. Although HIPAA contains some consumer protection components, the law basically creates a structure for the federal government to further regulate the operations of health plans. A positive feature of HIPAA is that health plan regulation remains with the states. The law also alleviates the need for the federal government to create a new regulatory structure to monitor consumer protection activities. A major drawback of the law is that standards are written into federal statute and become difficult to adapt as the health care system changes.

Medicare

In an effort to strengthen its already stringent rules for its managed care contractors, the Medicare program issued new regulations regarding physician incentive plans, grievances, and appeals. These regulations contain beneficiary notification requirements about provider reimbursement and require a disenrollment survey of Medicare beneficiaries to determine why they chose to leave a plan. The new regulations also address concerns about the time period for appeals by instituting an expedited appeals standard. Under the expedited appeals process, a health plan has 72 hours to review the denial of care if the beneficiary is suffering from a life-threatening condition. The expedited appeals process is activated upon physician request, regardless of the severity of the case. Medicare is also examining the length of time allowed for standard appeals and is discussing a change from 60 to 30 days.

49

In addition to internal rules changes, Congress enacted some changes for Medicare managed care in the Balanced Budget Act of 1997, including:

- banning "gag" clauses in physician contracts;
- establishing a "prudent layperson" standard for emergency care; and
- codifying the expedited appeal rule.

President's Advisory Commission on Consumer Protection and Quality in the Health Care Industry

Concerns about consumer protection and health care quality prompted President Clinton to appoint a 32-member commission of consumer advocates, providers, and health plan executives. In November 1997, the commission issued its report and recommended several "rights":

1. The right of consumers to have certain information disclosed to them, including covered benefits, cost sharing, grievance and appeals procedures, and licensure and credentials of providers.
2. The right to a choice of providers.
3. The right to emergency services.
4. The right to disclosure of all treatment options (whether covered or noncovered benefits).
5. The right to nondiscrimination against consumers on the basis of race, gender, religion, sexual orientation, or mental or physical disability.
6. The right to confidentiality of health information.
7. The right to consumer responsibility, including maximizing healthy habits such as exercising, not smoking, and eating a healthy diet.

In February 1998, President Clinton issued an order for all federal health care programs, including Medicare, Medicaid, the Federal Employees Health Benefits Program, the Department of Defense, and the Department of Veterans Affairs, to comply with the commission's recommendations by December 1999.

■ Conclusion

Will we look back on 1998 as the year of the managed care consumer? Numerous states are enacting their own managed care consumer protection laws. On the federal level, President Clinton, in his State of the Union address, emphasized his plans to translate the recommendations of his health care quality commission into a bill, which has been introduced in Congress as the Patient's Bill of Rights Act of 1998.

■ Key Terms

Agency for Health Care
  Policy and Research
  (AHCPR)
Commonwealth
  Foundation Survey
  (1995)
Consumer protection
  laws
Foundation for
  Accountability
  (FACCT)

Health Insurance
  Portability and
  Accountability Act
  (HIPAA)
HEDIS data
Medical record
  confidentiality
  standards
National Association of
  Insurance
  Commissioners'
  (NAIC's) model acts

Polling data
President's Advisory
  Commission on
  Consumer Protection
  and Quality in the
  Health Care Industry
Consumer protection
  standards
State consumer
  protection laws

Section II

WHO ARE THE PURCHASERS OF MANAGED CARE?

The proven success of managed care as a means to control rising employer health care premiums attracts other purchasers of health care services. This section examines those new purchasers in the managed care marketplace, and updates information on buying trends among the federal and state governments and employer coalitions. Combined, these entities represent the largest purchasers of managed care services. They are the impetus for the growth of managed care across the nation and across economic and social lines.

Chapter 4 provides updated information on purchasing trends among public and private purchasing groups. Chapter 5 presents an overview of the Federal Employees Health Benefits Program's new managed care efforts. Chapter 6 is an overview of the TRICARE program, the Department of Defense's approach to managed care, one component of which replaces the CHAMPUS program. Chapter 7 describes Medicare's managed care effort, including its new Medicare+Choice program. Chapter 8 reviews how states use managed care to purchase health care services for Medicaid and other populations for which they are responsible.

Chapter 4

MANAGED CARE AND PUBLIC AND PRIVATE PURCHASING GROUPS

■ Introduction

In the early 1980s, employers turned to management approaches when rising health care costs plagued traditional indemnity insurance arrangements. These approaches mirror the activities initiated by the Health Care Financing Administration (HCFA) to implement new Medicare and Medicaid managed care options that were codified into law in 1982 (Tax Equity and Fiscal Responsibility Act of 1982—TEFRA). Prior to these TEFRA amendments, the only program addressing utilization management (except for sporadic HMO contracts) was the 1974 legislation that created professional standards review organizations (PSROs). The PSROs were local physician-run organizations under contract with HCFA to monitor the medical necessity, appropriateness, and quality of care provided to people who were eligible for Medicare and Medicaid. The PSROs' management approaches included utilization review for medical necessity and appropriateness, and medical care evaluation studies to monitor quality of care.

Employers and large insurance companies that serve national employer accounts (such as Aetna U.S. Healthcare and CIGNA) readily adopted the utilization review feature. Initially, insurers added utilization review to medical plans only at the direction of the employer purchaser. Once cost savings became evident, insurers incorporated utilization review approaches into their own lines of business. Large case management, "not ordered not delivered," and second opinions for surgery became commonplace.

■ The Employer as Purchaser

With limited resources, employers address health expenditures with the same management approaches used to handle the direct operating expenditures of their core business. In a shift from their historical role as payers to their new role as health care managers, most employers now monitor health care processes and treat health care purchasing as a management function. Some multisite employers allocate health care expenditures to local operating units and hold local plant managers and personnel directors financially accountable for health plan decisions and expenditures. This transfer of accountability from a corporate office function to a local management activity fuels the growth of local business groups or coalitions.

Health Care Purchasing as a Management Function

Employers continue to be responsible for a large portion of U.S. health care expenditures. This responsibility spurs some more sophisticated employers to monitor the appropriateness and quality of health care services through such avenues as accreditation by the National Committee for Quality Assurance (NCQA) and the Joint Commission on Accreditation of Health Care Organizations (JCAHO). In addition, employers arrange with groups such as the Foundation for Accountability (FACCT) and the Oregon Medical Professional Review Organization (OMPRO) to evaluate a sample of care provided to corporate health plan enrollees and their dependents.

Employers also demand more involvement in the measurement and monitoring of provider costs. In addition to per-day or per-discharge savings generated by the discounted fee approach of preferred provider organizations (PPOs), employers want stable, multiyear protection against excessive health cost escalation. Employers know that the managed care option saves money both on a per-enrollee basis and on annual price increases. In situations where providers or health plans fail to create cost containment initiatives acceptable to employers, the employers may seek to save money through the development of their own health care delivery systems.

The Individual Employer

Most employer-sponsored managed care initiatives have been generated by large corporations, which are perceived to have the flexibility to self-insure and to obtain benefits from state benefit mandates. In self-insuring or self-funding, large employers avoid the premium taxes and risk charges associated with insured products. These large employers direct health plans to effectively control costs across their entire employee base, leading to health care cost management approaches that reach well beyond traditional utilization review/management. Employers expect processes to manage care when a health care encounter occurs, and to anticipate use of resources. This anticipation of resource usage gave rise to the popularity of "disease management" programs among large employers.

Smaller Employers as Purchasers

Smaller employers are able to take advantage of many of the approaches used by large employers, but often lack the staff knowledge or time to perform the required investigation. Without government or grant seed money, or sponsorship by a local big business coalition, small employer purchasing groups find it difficult to attract the resources (time and money) from businesses in which the owner wears many hats or those that lack a full-time benefits manager. To overcome these obstacles, San Francisco insurance brokers fashioned a "Benefits Alliance" (BA) for employers with 50–2,000 employees. California employers with fewer than 50 employees can access the negotiating and purchasing expertise of the Health Insurance Plan of California. By combining resources, these smaller California employers can afford expert consultants, an advantage that is likely beyond the reach of a single small employer.

Collective Employer Efforts

Employers use a number of approaches to encourage health care providers to make changes in their operational structures. The most common approach is the collective purchasing arrangement. This arrangement concentrates the purchasing power of small- and medium-sized employers—the demand-side of the health care equation. The goal of such collective purchasing arrangements is usually to contract with a risk-bearing organization for a new type of tightly managed coverage, to include:

■ premium rates based on risk-pooling among a large number of employers;

■ rates guaranteed for three years;

■ guaranteed acceptance of all of an employer's insured individuals;

■ risk-sharing with hospitals and physicians; and

■ performance measures based on medical outcomes, patient satisfaction, and service levels.

A number of cities (Minneapolis, Milwaukee, Denver, Memphis, Orlando, and Seattle) have successfully established collective employer purchasing arrangements.

Other Potential Purchasing Groups

Health benefit trusts—which have not yet entered the purchasing sphere in any large way—are potentially powerful purchasers. The trusts often combine labor and management and may include worker representatives who voice very specific health care system needs.

Health benefit trusts are typically organized as Voluntary Employees' Beneficiary Associations (VEBAs) and incorporated as nontaxable corporations [IRC 501 (c)(9)]. The Employee Retirement Income Security Act (ERISA) defines a multi-employer plan as a single plan contributed to by one or more unrelated employers pursuant to collective bargaining agreements. The Labor Management Relations Act of 1947 (Taft-Hartley Act), amending the National Labor Relations Act of 1935, provides for the establishment of trusts to offer health benefits to employees whose benefits are collectively bargained.

Taft-Hartley Trusts, Multiple Employer Trusts (METs), and Multiple Employer Welfare Associations (MEWAs)

METs and MEWAs are usually groups of small employers that join together (by nature of their business or regional location) to offer co-developed health benefit plans to their employees. Grouping helps small employers obtain better premiums because of the size of the combined group. Some METs and MEWAs even become funded organizations.

Taft-Hartley trusts result from collective bargaining between employers and labor representatives. Employers contribute to a trust to provide employee benefits to participants and beneficiaries of the trust. These trusts are regulated by federal law and managed by a joint board of trustees with equal representation of employer and labor. The trustees accept a fiduciary obligation to manage the trust and its assets in the best interests of the participants and beneficiaries.

The Taft-Hartley trusts are collectively bargained. The amount an employer contributes reflects a choice made by employees, through their labor representatives, to allocate a portion of a total compensation package as health benefits in lieu of wages. Under this form of "collective" rather than "individual" decision making, union members define contract goals and make negotiating decisions. The process educates the representatives of the union as they listen to employer arguments for less-expensive plans. Understanding health benefits costs, the representatives can judge if the benefits in a more costly package are worth the wages deferred to cover the premium cost. Their decisions are put to a vote in a contract ratification procedure.

As employee representatives gain an equal vote on the joint board of trustees, the overall design of these health benefit plans reflects the features negotiated (and paid for by the employees in deferred wages) through the collective bargaining process. This accountability for cost and plan design is central to the management and administration of a Taft-Hartley trust. It provides strong incentives for the trustees to minimize administrative expenses by:

■ permitting a greater percentage of each dollar to be used for health benefits;

■ including cost control and managed care features within plan designs; and

■ offering participant education programs.

On the other hand, because the trust exists to provide health benefits for employees represented by the labor organization, eligibility and coverage rules are liberal and flexible. This situation reflects the unique problem encountered in various industries covered by Taft-Hartley trusts. However, the unique features of these trusts may lend themselves to collective purchasing arrangements.

Partnerships

While health care purchasing arrangements often focus on financial or cost aspects, a growing trend for purchasers is to measure both customer and clinical service parameters. When clinical parameters and quality of care and services are considered, collective purchasing arrangements may involve health plans, other payers, providers, practitioners, and even the community as participants.

Health Plans and Other Reimbursement Partners

Employer collective purchasing arrangements may link up with a health plan or plans to offer benefits in certain geographic areas. The health plan usually agrees to terms specified by the collective purchasing arrangement. Such terms often include performing clinical quality studies, producing data reports, and setting costs over a period of (usually) three years. The health plan gains the right to put on a "health fair" in the workplace where employees can review the plan with a in-person representative, rather than only through printed materials. Health plan marketing experts believe that such one-on-one contacts are the best way to reach future plan participants.

Provider Partners

In some areas, especially smaller or rural communities, employers often partner with a specific group of health care providers. The providers agree to the requirements of the employer group. They may be organized as a physician hospital organization (PHO) or a physician hospital community organization (PHCO). Small or rural area employers can thus contract for care collectively with a single entity. Employers expect to gain managed care benefits since the PHOs and PHCOs usually act as an MCO or contract for the managed care functions.

Communitywide Efforts

Another emerging trend is community involvement in employer collective purchasing efforts. The logic behind employers' interest in the community stems from the fact that it is the source of the work force. The healthier the community, the healthier the potential employees. The better the community's ability to deal with issues such as teen pregnancy, diabetes, asthma, and cardiac conditions, the more likely it is that the employer will be able to manage health care expenditures.

The group most often involved at the community level is the local health department or local health jurisdiction. It has the skills and resources to provide health care services to all members of the community and has access to communitywide health demographics. One innovative example exists in the state of Washington, where, in a number of communities, local health departments joined forces with nearby hospitals and physicians to address communitywide health services and health management. That arrangement is rare, however; more common are public/private partnerships (e.g., as found in Minnesota) or public buy-ins to private coalitions (e.g., Children's Health Initiative Program).

■ Employer Coalitions

Business coalitions on health began in the late 1970s. Many grew out of local chamber of commerce efforts to address employer frustration with the increasing cost of health insurance premiums. Typically, large employers initiated these coalitions as a forum to discuss escalating health care costs, differences among employer health insurance plans, and local delivery system issues. Many early coalitions worked cooperatively with government-sponsored health system agencies (HSAs) charged with evaluating the need for new health care services, hospital beds, and capital building projects. Remnants of this initial effort are noted today when business and hospitals jointly lobby state legislatures to regulate the growth of freestanding health care facilities.

Early in the coalition movement, employers invited providers, insurers, and other interest groups to work cooperatively on the issues affecting employer health care benefits. Different agendas slowed progress and resulted in employer-only coalitions or business groups on health. As more employer-only groups emerged, they set specific work plans for collective purchasing, quality management, information systems, and legislative advocacy.

Employer efforts met with varying degrees of success. Companies with a large potential liability (a large work force) and adequate human resource staff succeeded more often than smaller or leaner employers. The role of business coalitions gained the attention of corporate CEOs around the country when it became obvious to their benefits managers that the federal government's ratcheting down of reimbursement for Medicare and contributions to Medicaid had resulted in a cost shift to private purchasers and contributed to premium inflation. Once it was clear how health care costs impact wages, that reality roused the ire of labor unions, affected domestic and international competitiveness, and created havoc with corporate balance sheets as accounting rules changed. With the stakes too high to continue in a business-as-usual mode, the coalition movement arrived at its second crossroads. A new community-based, market-oriented model for health care reform emerged, spearheaded by empowered employers willing to "buy-right" by dealing directly with hospitals, physicians, and other service providers to improve medical quality and cost-effectiveness.

National Coalitions

The Washington Business Group on Health (WBGH) and the National Business Coalition on Health (NBCH) are two well-known national employer coalitions.

- The Washington Business Group on Health began in the late 1970s and is the only national nonprofit organization devoted exclusively to the analysis of health policy and related work site issues from the perspective of large employers. Typically composed of Fortune 500 and large public sector employers, WBGH members are innovative health care purchasers that provide health coverage for more than 39 million U.S. workers, retirees, and their families.

- The National Business Coalition on Health started in the late 1980s to represent member coalitions that meet these criteria:
  - are not-for-profit groups;
  - have a majority of board members representing non-provider employers;
  - are commited to the concept of local community-based, market-driven health care reform.

More than 70 employer coalitions, representing over 5,000 employers and 20 million employees and dependents around the United States, are now members.

Regional, State, and Local Employer Coalitions

The coalition's number of members and importance to the local economy often determine its relative market clout. The more covered lives in a coalition (or if a community's most influential and largest employer participates), the more market power or perceived market power the coalition wields.

Participation by a state employee benefit plan or Medicaid program enhances a coalition's impact because of the additional volume and because the involvement of the government appeals to most providers. Employer coalitions with state government members include:

- Pacific Business Group on Health with the state of California (CALPERS); and
- Buyers Health Care Action Group (BHCAG), in Minneapolis, with state of Minnesota employees.

Other local employer groups achieve market presence without government involvement on a local level. For example,

- Gateway Purchasing Association in St. Louis represents 10 percent of the St. Louis market.
- Community Health Purchasing Corporation in Des Moines is a coalition of nine large, local employers that represents 20 percent of the area's private sector employees.

At the local level, the saying, "If you have seen one employer, you have seen one employer" is a proven truth. Each community, its employers, and its health care services are different. Employer coalitions differ in their expectations of how work is defined and carried out in each community.

Coalition Activities

Today, most coalitions center their activities around purchasing arrangements, quality measurement, and documentation of change in the delivery of health care services. Some examples are:

- The Washington Business Group on Health focuses on mental illness and disability issues, with an interest in health care and employee productivity.
- The National Business Coalition on Health assists individual coalition members with collective purchasing and quality measurement. Individual member coalitions usually select one key project, such as collective purchasing or a telephone advice system (Rochester, NY). Other projects may involve a quality-of-care study of an illness such as diabetes, or individual employer members may focus on a health care condition such as breast cancer.

■ Texas employers interested in collective purchasing initiated a new approach whereby employers in an area work together to control health care expenditures and the enterprise that manages the collective purchasing activity receives a percentage of the saving realized or negotiated that year.

Coalition Continuity

A critical measure of a coalition's success is its staying power. Very few business coalitions survive when key coalition staff leave, especially those who successfully and aggressively positioned the coalition. The dynamics of a coalition may create a need for self-reinvention (e.g., The Ozarks Business Group on Health, The South Florida [Miami] Coalition, The Texas Business Group on Health all exist, but in different forms than originally). Some coalitions exist only on paper, while others are "lunch and discussion" groups that rarely are aggressive purchasers. Still other coalitions emerge from restructuring and are highly successful. For example, the Minnesota Business Group on Health dissolved, only to reform and emerge as the Buyers Health Care Action Group. The reorganized group is now composed of only large employers and is a serious purchaser of health services.

Health care coalitions cannot rest on their accomplishments. They must evolve to best represent the interests of their employer members. The marketplace and U.S. demographics demand that coalitions find solutions to new issues such as productivity and health, the older worker, and health needs of retirees.

■ Conclusion

Most coalitions' efforts have concentrated on collective purchasing and study topics related to the current work force, such as C-section rates, asthma, diabetes, back pain, and depression. Emphasis has been on the management of the acute phase of an illness with guidelines and clinical pathways, with more recent attention on disease management.

In the future, coalitions must address new issues. The retiree population is increasing because of the early retirements that result from corporate "rightsizing" and because members of the baby boom generation are beginning to reach retirement age. With many employers responsible for retiree health benefits, coalitions need to place more attention on health management along the entire continuum of care, including preventive care and both functional and health risk status activities.

■ Key Terms

Accreditation

Business groups/ coalitions

Buyers Health Care Action Group (BHCAG) in Minneapolis

Coalition continuity

Collective purchasing

Community Health Purchasing Corporation in Des Moines, Iowa

Employer coalitions

Foundation for Accountability (FACCT)

Gateway Purchasing Association in St. Louis

Health Care Financing Administration (HCFA)

Health Insurance Plan of California (HIPC)

Joint Commission on Accreditation of Health Care Organizations (JCAHO)

Multiple Employer Trusts (METs)

Multiple Employer Welfare Association (MEWA)

National Business Coalition on Health (NBCH)

National Committee for Quality Assurance (NCQA)

Pacific Business Group on Health (PBGH)

Partnerships

Professional Standards Review Organizations (PSROs)

Quality monitoring

Small employer

Taft-Hartley trusts

Tax Equity and Fiscal Responsibility Act of 1982 (TEFRA)

Washington Business Group on Health (WBGH)

Chapter 5

THE FEDERAL EMPLOYEES HEALTH BENEFITS PROGRAM

■ Introduction

The Federal Employees Health Benefits (FEHB) Program, the largest employee benefits program of its kind, was established by an act of Congress, effective July 1, 1960. The FEHB Program now provides benefits to more than 9.5 million federal enrollees and dependents under contracts with approximately 350 carriers. The program covers most active, full-time civilian employees of the U.S. government, the U.S. Postal Service, and federal retirees (annuitants).

The U.S. Office of Personnel Management (OPM) administers the FEHB Program on behalf of more than 100 government agencies, the actual employers of FEHB enrollees, and federal retirement systems. Health plan contractors share responsibilities with the OPM and with federal agencies in carrying out the program. The OPM contracts for three types of health plans: (1) a governmentwide service benefit plan administered by the Blue Cross and Blue Shield Association; (2) employee organization plans sponsored by federal unions and other employee organizations; and (3) comprehensive medical plans, which are HMOs and other MCOs. Although only comprehensive medical plans initially offered managed care benefits, since 1990 all carriers participating in the FEHB Program have been required to implement substantial managed care operations.

The FEHB Program is authorized and operates under the FEHB Act (Chapter 89, title 5, United States Code) and FEHB Regulations (5 CFR Part 890). FEHB contracts must also conform with the Federal Acquisition Regulations (FAR) (48 CFR Ch. 1) in general and the Federal Employees Health Benefits Acquisition Regulations (FEHBAR) (48 CFR Ch. 16) in particular. The program is specifically exempt from the competitive bidding requirements of federal procurement law.

To carry out its role, the OPM contracts with private health plans on a calendar-year basis geared to the annual federal health benefits open season in November and December. Benefits and rates are negotiated between June and August each year and are effective in January of the following year. Each health plan's FEHB brochure is prepared in August and September, and the certified text is incorporated in the contract as the official statement of the plan's benefits; other contract provisions are uniform for all health plan contractors of similar type and rate structure. FEHB contracts are executed prior to the beginning of its contract year.

■ Unique FEHB Program Features

The FEHB Program is different from other employer-sponsored health programs. Beyond its sheer size, some major differences are:

Acceptance

Health plans must accept all federal employees or annuitants whose enrollments are certified by their agencies and who meet the plan's service and/or enrollment area requirements (as stated on the cover of the plan brochure), regardless of their age, health, or Medicare status.

Effective Dates

The effective date of an enrollment or an enrollment change is set by each enrollee's personnel office or retirement system, not by the plan. Enrollments and enrollment changes for employees typically do not become effective on the first of the month, but are tied to federal pay periods. Retiree enrollment changes usually are effective at the first of the month.

Enrollment Records

Employment and enrollment records for active federal employees are maintained by each employee's personnel office and not by the OPM. Therefore, OPM personnel cannot verify the enrollment of any active federal employee; only his or her personnel office can verify employment and enrollment. The OPM does not even maintain a list of the joint agency personnel offices and telephone numbers.

Insurance Officer

An insurance officer, often referred to as a health benefits officer, is responsible for administration of FEHB Program activities at each local agency or federal installation. The duties of the insurance officer are to explain the FEHB Program to employees, determine eligibility for enrollment, set the effective dates of health benefits actions, counsel employees on health benefits matters, and authorize on-site presentations or health fairs during open season.

Premiums

Health plans do not bill the OPM for premiums. Premium payments are based solely on the amount of funds collected from the individual payroll offices for a specific time period and are forwarded to the respective plans. Health plans receive premiums twice a month, in a lump sum, and the amount varies.

Members Lists

No list of members or payroll offices accompanies the payment. Therefore, the only record of payment for federal members to the health plan is the receipts or accounting records kept by each health plan.

■ Contract Administration

The steps and time frames to administer the FEHB Program are well defined.

The "Call Letter" and Rate/Benefit Negotiations

By March 31 of each calendar year, the OPM's Office of Insurance Programs issues its annual "Call Letter" to all participating carriers, outlining the major program objectives for the next contract year. Policy decisions regarding the scope of desired benefit changes and extent of permitted rate increases are discussed. May 31 is the regulatory deadline for plans to submit proposed benefit changes, service area expansions, and requests to add or eliminate rating areas. It is also the regulatory deadline for plans to submit their rate proposals for the next benefit year. June 30 is the deadline to submit documentation for service area expansions (e.g., state authorizations and provider contracts) and for state community benefits package approvals. During the months of June through August, the OPM and the plans negotiate rates, benefits, and service area proposals.

Annual "Open Season"

During the annual open season, employees may enroll in the FEHB Program and current enrollees may change their plan enrollments. After it reaches agreement with all contracting plans on rates and benefits for the ensuing benefit year, the OPM prepares the FEHB *Guide* and other open season material. The OPM issues a press release to announce the open season and FEHB rates for the coming year. A *Federal Register* notice, issued earlier, announces the specific open season dates, which occur from mid-November to mid-December.

■ Marketing and Servicing

Reaching Federal Workers and Annuitants

Each fall, the OPM issues a Benefits Administration Letter to all agency insurance officers that lists the names, addresses, service areas, and open season contact information for all plans in the program. During the marketing process, each plan deals solely with individual agencies, not with the OPM. As previously stated, the OPM does not maintain a list of personnel offices, addresses, or phone numbers, so each plan must develop its own list of agency contacts. Federal agencies do not provide plans with the names and addresses of their employees.

The status of the enrollee defines the marketing approach.

Active Employees

Each plan prints and delivers copies of its brochure to federal agencies for distribution. In each plan's service area, active federal employees are found at installations of various federal agencies and the U.S. Postal Service. Employees are approached either at their work sites or through the media, and the plans may participate in health fairs held at federal installations. Plans are also required to mail plan literature to each of their current federal subscribers detailing the following year's rate and benefits.

Annuitants

When federal employees retire with FEHB coverage, they are no longer easily accessible to a plan's marketing staff. The plan is required to mail a specified number of brochures to an OPM contractor for distribution to annuitants who request plan information. Annuitants request plan brochures directly from the

OPM's contractor and change their enrollment by telephone or by filling out a special enrollment form.

Each subsequent year that a plan participates in the program, it must send one brochure to each of its federal enrollees in addition to the brochures it sends to federal installations and to the OPM's contractor.

Service Area and Providers

It is extremely important to the OPM that each plan accurately manages its service and enrollment area to ensure that plan members have easy access to plan providers and to minimize inappropriate use of non-plan providers.

Plans are responsible to review each new enrollee's address and to verify that the member resides (and/or works) within the plan's approved enrollment area as described in the current brochure. Moreover, federal enrollees must rely on the provider information they receive from FEHB plans; in the event a plan-certified provider directory is no longer accurate by open season, a plan must provide correct information to prospective members who inquire about a specific provider's availability in the upcoming year.

Complaints and Disputes

The OPM directs all written complaints or inquiries from enrollees to the plan and requests a copy of any written correspondence from the plan to the member. Written complaints are reviewed by the OPM contract specialist assigned to the plan.

Each plan must inform the enrollee of his or her right to an OPM review if the plan, upon reconsideration, upholds its initial denial of health benefits. Enrollees may bring disputes concerning benefits or services to the OPM for review after asking for reconsideration and failing to obtain a satisfactory reply. These disputed claims are reviewed within the OPM contracting division to which the plan is assigned. The OPM determines whether the enrollee or family member is entitled to the service or supply under the terms of the contract, as set forth in the brochure.

The OPM considers that a request for its review of a disputed claim constitutes authorization for the release of related medical information. By regulation, the plan must respond within 30 days to the OPM's request for information. Within 30 days after receiving all evidence, the OPM notifies both the plan and the claimant of its decision: either affirming the denial or instructing the plan to pay the claim or provide the service. Any litigation regarding a disputed claim decision by the OPM is initiated in a federal district court with the OPM as the defendant.

Cancellation and Termination

Under FEHB law, an enrollee may cancel his or her FEHB enrollment at any time, and government agencies may terminate coverage when the enrollee is no longer eligible. Under no circumstances, including fraud, may carriers terminate a federal enrollee. Only federal agencies are empowered to take disciplinary actions, including termination of employment, against employees who violate federal laws or standards of conduct.

Enrollment Reconciliations and Underpayments

The periodic reconciliation of enrollment records is required by each plan's contract with the OPM. Unfortunately, FEHB enrollment and payroll functions are performed by more than 700 personnel and payroll offices in many separate agencies. Therefore, the OPM is not in a position to reconcile carrier and government enrollment records. The OPM's role in the reconciliation process is to help carriers obtain the cooperation they need from the various agencies to reconcile any differences that they identify. To this end, the OPM issues guidelines to all FEHB carriers for reconciling enrollment records. The guidelines stress carrier contact with agency payroll/personnel officers because reconciliation problems are resolved at that level. The guidelines also request that the OPM receive detailed documentation of carrier actions in the event that intervention becomes necessary (e.g., if a payroll office does not provide requested information).

To assist with reconciliation, the OPM periodically issues a Headcount Report. This report provides a count of enrollments by payroll offices for the last payroll paid during the 1st through the 15th of March and September. In addition, each payroll office sends plans a quarterly report. This report includes enrollment data for the last payroll period (the 1st through the 15th of the last month in each quarter). This list of enrollee names and total money (withholdings and contributions) provides help to reconcile the plans' and the agency's enrollment data.

The OPM's Office of Retirement Programs provides the names, addresses, and other key annuitant information to carriers once a year, within two or three months after the March 31 semi-annual Headcount Report is released.

In 1997, the OPM instituted a new one percent loading to the premiums for participating plans to compensate for historic underpayments resulting from the inability of the plans to achieve complete reconciliation within the FEHB Program structure. Underpayments occur for a variety of reasons but generally result from the payroll offices' failure to report enrollment changes in a timely manner.

■ Rate Setting, Payment, and Audit

The FEHB Program Act and Regulations permit the OPM to contract with private health plans on either an experience-rated or a community-rated basis.

Community Rating

Community rating in the FEHB Program is a prospective rating method with various forms:

- ■ Traditional Community Rating (TCR) bases the rate for each group on an underlying communitywide capitation (per member/per month) rate.
- ■ Community Rating by Class (CRC) allows rate adjustments based on the age/sex distribution of each group.
- ■ Adjusted Community Rating (ACR) allows the use of the experience of the particular group to prospectively set rates.

The OPM purchases a plan's most popular "community benefits package" and adjusts it during negotiations. The health plan submits its rate proposal seven months before the rates take effect, so the proposed FEHB Program rate typically is based on an estimated community rate. The OPM performs a reconciliation before setting the next year's rate to ensure that the premium rate for the current year is based on the plan's actual community rate. The reconciliation is a re-submission of the current year's proposal, using the actual community rate instead of the estimated rate.

The OPM establishes a contingency reserve for each plan by adding a three percent increment to the premium negotiated with each plan. The contingency reserve funds represent equity of the FEHB Program, not the carrier, and are used for the benefit of the enrollees who contributed them. These funds, set aside for the plan, cannot contribute to the health plan's solvency or offset plan costs. However, through the reconciliation process, the contingency reserve can reimburse plans for money owed by the government.

Experience Rating

Experience rating in the FEHB Program is retrospective. The premium is based on the specific claims of the health plan's federal enrollees. Experience rating in the FEHB Program assumes that any excess of premium over obligations and agreed-upon profit with respect to the federal group is returned to the group or held for the group's benefit. The premium is adjusted annually based on the amount of the contingency reserves the OPM holds for each plan, the accrued claims reserve, and the positive or negative difference between income and expenses.

Experience-rated plans may receive a profit referred to as a "service charge." The service charge is determined by a weighted guidelines method in which the OPM applies several factors to projected incurred claims and allowable administrative expenses:

■ carrier's performance;

■ share of cost risk;

■ efforts at advancing federal socioeconomic programs;

■ capital investments not allowable as administrative expenses;

■ efforts to control costs; and

■ independent development that is of demonstrated value to the FEHB Program.

The OPM does not guarantee a minimum service charge. Costs allowable under an experience-rated contract are the actual, necessary, and reasonable amounts incurred, as determined in accordance with the contract, the Federal Acquisition Regulation, and Federal Employees Health Benefits Acquisition Regulation. Contract costs consist of benefit costs and administrative costs.

Government Contributions

The maximum amount that the government contributes toward the cost of health benefits is determined each year, in accordance with the FEHB Act. Through 1998, the act specifies that the government shall pay 60 percent of the number determined by averaging the rates of specified large plans representing the three categories of plans in the FEHB Program. Beginning in 1999, the government contribution increases to 72 percent of the weighted average of premiums for all plans for self-only and for self-and-family coverage. The government contribution is not more than 75 percent of the total premium of any one plan, with one exception: The U.S. Postal Service contribution can go higher, in accordance with prevailing labor agreements.

Audits and SSSGs

The OPM Office of the Inspector General (OIG) periodically audits all carriers. The emphasis of the audit varies, depending on the type of carrier.

Community Rating

Community-rated carriers' records are reviewed to determine whether the rate charged to the FEHB Program was developed according to the contract, the FAR, and the FEHBAR. Routine audits consist of two types: (1) a historical audit that generally covers five contract years, and (2) a rate reconciliation audit that covers only the current year's proposed rate reconciliation. Both types of audits analyze the plan's methodology and supporting documentation underlying the federal premium rates, including the special benefits and loadings. The audit emphasizes verification that the plan's federal rate is consistent with the rates charged to the plan's two "similarly sized subscriber groups" (SSSGs), as defined in the FEHBAR.

The OPM requires contractors to rate the FEHB Program in accordance with the same methodology (including discounts) used in rating the plan's SSSGs. Every group of a plan is a potential SSSG. The term includes groups enrolled in a separate line of business of the contractor, governmental accounts, and groups that purchase a point-of-service product. The only exceptions are groups that are retrospectively experience-rated, groups consisting of the plan's own employees, Medicare and Medicaid groups, and groups that purchase only a single benefit (such as dental benefits) from the carrier. Each community-rated plan submits an annual Certificate of Accurate Pricing. This document certifies to the OPM that the program's rates were developed by the contractor with the same methodology used for the two SSSGs. If an audit determines that one or both SSSGs received a rate advantage (i.e., discount) not given to the FEHB Program, then the contractor's certificate is classified "defective" and a financial penalty is assessed. Under some circumstances, the OIG will refer the audit to the U.S. Attorney's Office for investigation of possible violations of the False Claims Act.

Experience Rating

Financial and claims records are reviewed to determine whether an experience-rated carrier charged expenses to the contract in accordance with the contract, the FAR, and the FEHBAR. Specific review areas may include coordination of benefits, cost containment efforts, economy and efficiency reviews, and determination that costs are allowable, allocable, and reasonable.

All audits include carrier fraud and abuse detection and prevention procedures, as well as a review of internal controls.

■ Conclusion

The FEHB Program has served as a model for employer-sponsored health insurance programs, in part because of its size and in part because it embodies the principles of managed competition that figure prominently in recent health care reform discussions. However, the program is becoming more regulated, as demonstrated by the SSSG-based audits of community-related plans—the OPM's unique approach to preventing fraud against the federal government. The broad definition of an SSSG requires all FEHB Program participants to prepare commercial rates with one eye toward passing approval under the FEHBAR audit standards.

Advocates of market competition are expected to continue efforts to experiment with the FEHB Program. Already, legislation has been introduced to add a Medical Savings Account option to the program.

Studies suggest that increased efficiency can be achieved by reducing the number of plans, particularly comprehensive plans, that participate in the FEHB Program. It is unclear whether such studies will trigger the introduction of a competitive bidding process into the FEHB Program.

■ Key Terms

Adjusted Community
  Rating (ACR)
Annual "open season"
Annuitants
Benefits Administration
  Letter
"Call Letter"
Cancellation,
  termination
Community rating
Community rating by
  class (CRC)

Complaints
Enrollment records
Enrollments,
  reconciliations,
  underpayments
Experience rating
Federal Acquisition
  Regulations
  (FAR)
Federal Employees
  Health Benefits
  (FEHB) Program

Federal Employees
  Health Benefits
  Acquisition
  Regulations (FEHBAR)
Headcount Report
Insurance officer
Office of Personnel
  Management (OPM)
Office of the Inspector
  General (OIG)
OPM Office of
  Retirement Programs

Rate/benefit
negotiationsService
charge

Similarly sized
subscriber groups
(SSSGs)

Chapter 6

TRICARE: A MANAGED CARE OPTION

■ Introduction

The Department of Defense's (DOD) primary health care mission is the maintenance of the health of 1.6 million active-duty personnel and the provision of
care during military operations. As an employer, the DOD offers health care to
6.6 million beneficiaries, including active duty personnel and their dependents
and military retirees and their dependents. The $15 billion Defense Health Pro-
gram accounts for about six percent of the DOD's total budget.

Most of the health care services rendered within the Department of Defense
are provided in approximately 115 hospitals and 470 clinics, referred to as Military Treatment Facilities (MTFs). They exist worldwide and are operated by the
Army, Navy, and Air Force. The DOD's direct care system is assisted or supple-
mented by health care services provided in civilian facilities but paid for by the
DOD. The General Accounting Office estimated that DOD expenses in fiscal
year 1997 were $12 billion to provide direct care to beneficiaries and $3.5 bil-
lion to provide care in civilian facilities.

■ TRICARE Implementation

In late 1993, the DOD launched TRICARE, a nationwide managed care program
intended to improve the military community's access to health care, maintain
quality, and control the $15 billion in annual health care expenditures. While
direct care is provided by DOD personnel in DOD facilities, the DOD's new
TRICARE program also includes direct health care provided by managed care
support contractors.

Table 6.1

TRICARE Five-Year Contracts Awarded by DOD (as of 6/98)

DOD Regions	Contractor	Amount
11 Northwest	Foundation Health Federal Services	$652 million
6 Southwest	Foundation Health Federal Services	$1.8 billion
9, 10, 12 California & Hawaii	Foundation Health Federal Services	$2.5 billion
3 and 4 Southeast & Gulf south	Human Military Healthcare Services	$3.8 billion
7 and 8 Central & Desert states	Trimmest Healthcare Alliance	$2.3 billion
2 National capital	Sierra Military Health Services	$1.213 million

TRICARE is a triple option program:

■ TRICARE Prime: a health maintenance organization (HMO)

■ TRICARE Extra: a preferred provider organization (PPO)

■ TRICARE Standard: a fee-for-service program (the former CHAMPUS program)

TRICARE operates in partnership with civilian contractors. Its goals are to:

■ ensure high-quality consistent health care benefits;

■ preserve beneficiaries' choice of health care providers;

■ improve access to care; and

■ contain health care costs.

To begin implementation of TRICARE throughout its 12 worldwide regions, the DOD issued seven large contracts that cover the seven TRICARE regions located in the United States.

The DOD lacks military-owned or -operated facilities that are geographically accessible to directly serve every beneficiary. To meet its health care obligations, the DOD contracts on a regional basis with civilian providers and networks to deliver the health care services. The civilian managed care contractors under TRICARE are required to assist in delivery of health care services and to provide administrative support that includes utilization review, case management, enrollment, and member services. The managed care contractor may also provide mail order pharmacy and mental health services. Regardless of the services provided, each managed care support contract is designed to support the basic military health care systems and jointly bring the TRICARE option to each DOD region. By June 1998, DOD had awarded TRICARE five-year contracts (one year with four option years) as shown in Table 6.1.

Active-duty beneficiaries are given priority for health care services in military-owned and -operated facilities. Retirees and their dependents over age 65 are

Table 6.2

Tricare Options

	Standard	Extra	Prime
Deductibles	Yes: the same as TRICARE	Yes; the same as TRICARE Standard	No, if care is received at an MTF or from civilian network
Cost shares or copayments	Yes; highest of all options	Yes; but 5% lower than TRICARE Standard	No, for care in MTF; nominal for civilian network care
Enrollment fees	None	None	No, for active duty families; yes, for retirees and their families
Out-of-pocket costs	Highest of all options	Lower than TRICARE Standard	No, for care in MTF (and far less than Standard and Extra for civilian network care)
Access to civilian doctors and hospitals	Greatest flexibility to choose a doctor and medical facility	Choice limited to network of civilian doctors	All care is provided through assigned primary care manager. Needed care not available at an MTF will be referred to civilian network.
Paper-filing claims for reimbursement	Sometimes	None	None
Preventive test/ exams	With applicable deductibles and copays	With applicable deductibles and copays	Recommended as part of primary care and included free of charge.
Primary care managers	No	No	Yes, key feature of this option

not eligible for TRICARE enrollment because they receive Medicare benefits. However, these seniors may receive care in DOD medical facilities on a space-available basis.

TRICARE beneficiaries may select one of the three managed care options in the DOD's new TRICARE system. Benefits in each option vary, as do the costs of annual membership for a beneficiary and his or her dependents. Table 6.2 highlights some features and benefits of the TRICARE options.

■ TRICARE Issues

The DOD recognizes that many of its beneficiaries obtain health care coverage from the private sector after retirement. These dual-eligibles are often referred to as "ghosts," a reference to beneficiaries eligible for DOD-sponsored programs but who choose private health care options for primary coverage. The DOD is

79

concerned about the heavy impact on the DOD system should a large number of "ghosts" discontinue their private coverage in favor of the DOD managed care option.

The DOD projects that a shift in those eligible for its health care coverage will occur in the following ways:

- Decrease in numbers
  Among active-duty personnel and their dependents, the DOD projects a two percent decrease between fiscal years 1997 and 2003, from 48 to 46 percent.
- Increase in numbers
  For retirees and their dependents, the DOD estimates a two percent increase, from 52 to 54 percent, over the same period. The Office of Health Affairs within the DOD expects the number of military retirees over the age of 65 to increase through the year 2014.

The issue of DOD retirees who are also covered by Medicare presents an ongoing problem between the Department of Defense and the Health Care Financing Administration (HCFA). As space in military treatment facilities becomes available to the over–65 retiree, the DOD has requested reimbursement from Medicare funds for these duly eligible persons. An amendment in the Balanced Budget Act of 1997 authorized six sites for a Medicare managed care demonstration subvention project between the two agencies. Under this demonstration project, the Department of Defense is paid a reduced percentage of the Medicare+Choice reimbursement rate, in return for providing Medicare covered services to the duly eligible military retirees. Enrollment began in January 1998, with the first DOD managed care sites expected to offer health care services in February 1998.

■ Conclusion

Implementation of the TRICARE program was delayed by protests from some contractors during the award process, which made the contracting process unappealing to other vendors. For example, the Region II contract was awarded, the award was protested and, with the protest upheld, the result was a new "best and final offer" process. This complex process slows down the target dates for the program and costs both the government and bidders additional funds.

The DOD is aware that its TRICARE contracts are large in scope and require compliance with cumbersome regulations. Discussions are under way to consider the possibility of contracting for managed care support on a local rather than regional basis and to allow private plans to "sell" their existing programs without the constraint of additional government regulations.

TRICARE is still too new to evaluate its success in accomplishing its mission: to improve access to and quality of health care services while containing costs.

■ Key Terms

Department of Defense
(DOD)
"Ghosts"

Medicare managed care
demonstration project
Military Treatment
Facility (MTF)

TRICARE Extra
TRICARE Prime
TRICARE Standard

Chapter 7

MANAGED CARE IN MEDICARE

◾ Introduction

Since 1992, Medicare and Medicaid beneficiary enrollment in managed care plans has experienced unprecedented growth. Although Medicaid is a combined federal and state program, growth in both programs makes the Health Care Financing Administration (HCFA) the largest purchaser of managed care in the country, accounting for about 19 million Americans. HCFA is expanding the choices for Medicare beneficiaries and working to ensure that all beneficiaries enrolled in managed care plans receive quality care.

As of January 1, 1997, more than 4.9 million Medicare beneficiaries were enrolled in a total of 336 managed care plans that account for 13 percent of the total Medicare population. This represents a 108 percent increase in Medicare managed care enrollment since 1993. In 1996, an average of 80,000 Medicare beneficiaries voluntarily enrolled in risk-bearing HMOs each month. Medicare beneficiaries may enroll or disenroll in a managed care plan at any time, and for any reason, with only 30 days' notice. However, that will change soon under recent amendments.

In general, Medicare beneficiaries may experience lower out-of-pocket costs and added coverage when they choose a prepaid Medicare participating health care plan (referred to as a "risk" plan) instead of receiving covered services under the Medicare program's traditional fee-for-service arrangements. Most Medicare beneficiaries live in areas served by at least one Medicare risk plan.

HCFA contracts with risk plans through a process that evaluates solvency, organizational structure, and the risk applicant's capabilities, along with its Medicare delivery system, to provide or arrange for the provision of covered benefits. If the plan is approved, HCFA pays the plan a fixed amount per member, per month (known as the AAPCC [adjusted average per capita cost]) for all Medicare-covered benefits. To attract beneficiaries, and depending on the rates available from the federal government, many MCOs offer additional benefits not covered by Medicare, such as routine eye examinations, pharmacy benefits, physical examinations, and routine office visits.

■ Medicare+Choice Program (Medicare Part C)

Public Law 105–33, the Balanced Budget Act of 1997 (BBA '97), enacted August 5, 1997, dramatically expands the options for Medicare beneficiaries. This legislation creates a new Medicare Part C program (also known as Medicare+Choice). The following description is based on information available from HCFA in early 1998.

Contracts with Medicare+Choice Plans

BBA '97 establishes a new authority that permits contracts between HCFA and a variety of different managed care and fee-for-service entities. The types of entities that may be granted contracts under this new authority include:

Coordinated Care Plans

Plans that include health maintenance organizations (HMOs), preferred provider organizations (PPOs), and provider-sponsored organizations (PSOs). A PSO is defined as a public or private entity established by health care providers that provides a substantial proportion of health care items and services directly through affiliated providers who share, directly or indirectly, substantial financial risk.

Religious, Fraternal Benefit Society Plans

Plans that may restrict enrollment to members of the church, convention, or group with which the society is affiliated. Payments to such plans may be adjusted, as appropriate, to take into account the actuarial characteristics and experience of plan enrollees.

Private Fee-for-Service Plans

Plans that reimburse providers on a fee-for-service basis and are authorized to charge enrolled beneficiaries up to 115 percent of the plan's payment schedule (which may differ from the Medicare fee schedule).

Medical Savings Account (MSA)

In addition to Medicare+Choice contractors, BBA '97 creates a Medical Savings Account (MSA) demonstration project. Beginning in January 1999 and ending January 1, 2003, a maximum of 390,000 Medicare beneficiaries can enroll in an MSA option. Under this option, Medicare beneficiaries obtain high deductible health policies that pay at least all Medicare-covered items and services, after an enrollee meets an annual deductible of up to $6,000. The difference between the premiums paid for an MSA policy and the Medicare+Choice premium amount is placed into an account for the beneficiary to use to meet his or her deductible expenses.

Current 1876 Contracts

HMOs or Competitive Risk Plans (CRPs) that comply with current HCFA contracting standards and with the new requirements established under BBA '97 automatically transition to the Medicare+Choice program. Since January 1, 1998, Section 1876 risk-based contractors are paid under a new Medicare+Choice payment methodology, rather than the current AAPCC method in Section 1876(a), and are subject to other Medicare+Choice provisions. Contracting standards for Medicare+Choice plans (except for PSO solvency standards) are to be published by June 1, 1998, as interim final regulations, and new Section 1876 risk applications are no longer accepted. As of January 1, 1999, existing Section 1876 risk-based contracts are terminated and plans in good standing transition to the Medicare+Choice program.

Repeal of Cost Option

As of August 5, 1997 (the date of enactment of the act), the Department of Health and Human Services (DHHS) was prohibited from entering into any new Section 1876 cost-based contracts, unless the plan is a health care prepayment plan (HCPP) with an agreement under Section 1833 of the Social Security Act. The 1876 cost-based payment authority is repealed, and all existing cost contracts ultimately terminate on December 31, 2002.

Limited HCPP Option

On January 1, 1999, the DHHS may only contract with those HCPPs that are sponsored by union or employer groups or that do not "provide, or arrange for the provision of, any inpatient hospital services. . .." This amendment terminates the 1833 agreements with any organization that fails to meet the new definition. HCFA must establish transition rules for Section 1876 risk-based contractors that currently are reimbursed on a cost basis for those enrollees who remain under a previous HCPP agreement.

1876 Contracting Option for PSOs

During the transition, PSOs that otherwise are eligible to obtain a Medicare risk contract under the current Section 1876 may do so. State-licensed PSOs that apply for a risk contract are required to meet all applicable standards for Competitive Medical Plans, except that the minimum enrollment requirements are reduced or waived effective January 1, 1998.

Medicare Subvention

BBA '97 authorizes six sites for a Medicare managed care subvention demonstration between HCFA and the DOD. Under this demonstration, the DOD is paid a reduced percentage of the Medicare+Choice reimbursement rate to provide Medicare covered services to eligible military retirees who are also Medicare eligible. Enrollment is expected to begin in early 1998. The DOD selected the first managed care sites for the demonstration program in February 1998.

■ Medicare+Choice Requirements

The following summarizes the statutory provisions that establish new Medicare +Choice program requirements or amend existing contractual standards. New contractual standards apply to Section 1876 risk plans that transition to the Medicare+Choice program for the contract year that begins on January 1, 1999.

Eligibility, Enrollment, and Disenrollment Requirements

Beneficiary Eligibility

With minor exceptions, only beneficiaries entitled to Part A and enrolled in Part B are eligible to enroll in a Medicare+Choice plan that serves their geographic area. HCFA will promulgate rules to permit the continued enrollment of Part B-only enrollees in those Section 1876 risk-based plans that transition into the Medicare+Choice program.

According to draft rules, Medicare+Choice plans may allow a beneficiary who moves outside the geographic area served by a Medicare+Choice plan to remain enrolled in the plan. However, the enrollee must have reasonable access to the full range of covered services as part of the basic benefit package.

Special Information Campaign

During November 1998, the DHHS will conduct a national educational campaign to inform Medicare beneficiaries about the availability of new health care options and the enrollment process to select a new option. Current 1876 Medicare risk plans must accept new Medicare enrollments during this period.

Enrollment

Beginning in November 1999, the DHHS is scheduled to conduct an annual national educational and publicity campaign to inform eligible beneficiaries about their Medicare+Choice plan options. An individual's choice of plans becomes effective on January 1, 2000. Newly eligible enrollees who do not select a Medicare+Choice plan are deemed to have chosen the original Medicare fee-for-service option. An exception allows the DHHS to establish procedures under which "age-ins" (people already in a health care plan who choose to stay in the same plan, but under Medicare+Choice after becoming eligible for Medicare) enrolled in a contracting plan are deemed as electing the entity's Medicare+Choice plan. Any beneficiary enrolled in an 1876 plan as of December 31, 1998, is considered enrolled with that organization under the Medicare+Choice program, if the plan is granted a Medicare+Choice contract starting January 1, 1999.

Disenrollment

In 2002, beneficiaries enrolled in a Medicare+Choice coordinated care plan can disenroll from their elected plan option only once during the first six months of the year. Beneficiaries who enroll in a Medicare+Choice plan at the time they become eligible for Medicare are permitted to disenroll at any time during the first year of enrollment.

Beginning January 1, 2003—and only once during the first three months of the calendar year—beneficiaries may:

■ disenroll from a Medicare+Choice coordinated care plan and choose another plan;

■ leave Medicare fee-for-service to enroll in a Medicare+Choice plan; or

■ return to Medicare fee-for-service.

This new requirement effectively locks beneficiaries into their Medicare+Choice plan election for the remaining nine months of the year. Exceptions are available for enrollees under certain circumstances, such as if a:

- Medicare+Choice plan contract is terminated;
- beneficiary leaves the plan service area; or
- Medicare+Choice plan fails to provide covered benefits or is found to be improperly marketing the Medicare product. (Other conditions having to do with the performance of the plan—yet to be specified by the DHHS—will also make exceptions possible.)

Medicare+Choice plans may disenroll a Medicare beneficiary if an enrollee is disruptive to plan operations or fails to pay required premiums in a timely fashion.

Coordinated Open-Enrollment Period

In November 1999, the DHHS must hold the first annual coordinated open-enrollment period to allow eligible beneficiaries to enroll in Medicare+Choice plans. Medicare+Choice plans are required to submit comparative information to the DHHS.

Marketing Material Approval

If a Medicare+Choice plan's marketing materials are approved for one service area, they are deemed as approved in all of the plan's service areas. One exception applies to area-specific information. Medicare+Choice plans are prohibited from offering monetary incentives for enrolling or for completing any portion of the enrollment application.

■ Contracting Standards

By June 1, 1998, the DHHS must publish interim final regulations for Medicare +Choice organizations that establish standards based on existing requirements contained in Part 417 of the Public Health Title of the Code of Federal Regulations. All Medicare+Choice applications must undergo review for compliance with the new standards. Any 1876 risk plan that transitions to the Medicare +Choice option is required to meet the contracting standards for the contract year that begins January 1, 1999.

Federal standards preempt any state authority regarding benefit requirements for inclusion of, or treatment by, providers, and for coverage determinations, including related appeals and grievance processes.

Benefit Changes

Public Law 105–33 establishes some new Medicare preventive benefits and increases coverage for others. The updates to payment rates for current 1876 risk

Table 7.1

New Medicare Benefits and Effective Dates

Benefit	Effective date
Annual screening mammography (women over 40)	January 1, 1998
Screening PAP smear and pelvic exam (every 3 years)	January 1, 1998
Colorectal cancer screening exam	January 1, 1998
Bone density measurement (rules out osteoporosis)	July 1, 1998
Prostate cancer screening exam (men over 50)	January 1, 2000

contractors and Medicare+Choice plans must reflect the costs of these new Medicare benefits. The new benefits and effective dates are shown in Table 7.1.

Disclosure Rules

The Medicare+Choice plan must provide each enrollee, using a clear, accurate, and standardized form, with information about the plan's:

■ service area;

■ benefits;

■ number, mix, and distribution of providers;

■ out-of-area coverage;

■ emergency coverage;

■ supplemental benefits;

■ prior authorization rules;

■ appeals and grievance procedures; and

■ quality assurance program.

Upon request, enrollees must be provided with:

■ a comparison of the plan's benefits with traditional Medicare benefits;

■ a description of the plan's utilization review mechanisms;

■ information on the number of grievances and appeals the plan has experienced and their disposition in the aggregate; and

■ a summary of physician compensation arrangements.

Access to Non-Network Providers

Medicare+Choice plans must cover services of non-network providers for:

- medically necessary urgent care when the enrollee is out of the plan service area;
- renal dialysis services for enrollees who are temporarily outside the plan's service area; and
- maintenance or post-stabilization care after an emergency condition is stabilized.

Medicare+Choice plans are required to pay for emergency services regardless of prior authorization or the emergency provider's status as a network provider. "An emergency medical condition" is defined under the "prudent layperson" standard and may include the beneficiary's assertion of "severe pain."

Provider Participation

Medicare+Choice plans must establish procedures for physician participation in the plan, including notice of rules of participation, written notice of adverse participation decisions, and an appeals process. Medicare+Choice plans must consult with participating physicians regarding medical policy, quality, and medical management procedures.

Medicare+Choice plans are prohibited from requiring contracting providers to indemnify the plan against actions that result from the plan's denial of medically necessary care.

Plans may not restrict a health care professional's advice to an enrollee regarding health status or treatment options. BBA '97 includes a "conscience protection" clause that exempts a plan from requirements to provide or cover a counseling or referral service if the plan:

- objects on moral or religious grounds;
- informs prospective enrollees of such a policy before or during enrollment; or
- informs current enrollees within 90 days after adopting a change in such a policy.

Physician Incentive Rules

Since January 1997, plans are required to disclose financial incentives and purchase stop-loss insurance so that not more than 25 percent of a physician's income is at risk under capitation. The regulations also ban any incentive arrangements that include payments to doctors to limit or reduce medically necessary services for a specific patient. These rules are designed to ensure that incentives to discourage unnecessary services for a patient do not jeopardize quality.

▓ Payment Requirements

Announcement of the 1998 Medicare AAPCC payment rates for 1876 risk-based contracts and new Medicare+Choice plans occurred in September 1997. Starting in March 1998, the Medicare+Choice payment rates for the following contract year were announced. In general, the Medicare capitation rates are the greater of:

- a blend of the input-price adjusted national rate and an area-specific rate, adjusted by a budget neutrality factor. The area-specific rate is based on 1997 rates and is adjusted to reflect the national average Medicare per capita growth rate and the gradual removal of IME/GME (Indirect Medical Education/Graduate Medical Education) costs; and

- a minimum payment amount of $367 for 1998, not to exceed 150 percent of the prior year rate, adjusted annually by a defined update factor; or

- a minimum percentage increase (two percent per year).

The 1997 capitation rates (from the 1997 AAPCC rate book) provide the base for area-specific rates in the blend and minimum percentage increase rates. In an area where the 1997 AAPCC varies by more than 20 percent from the 1996 AAPCC, the DHHS can substitute a rate more indicative of the cost of Medicare-covered services for beneficiaries in the area. The update factor for the area-specific rates in the blend and the minimum payment amount is the national average per capita Medicare+Choice growth rate, reduced by 0.8 percentage points for 1998, 0.5 percentage points for 1999 through 2002, and 0.0 percentage points thereafter.

The payment area is the county or equivalent area specified by the DHHS. In 1999, states may request a statewide payment rate or a rate based on Metropolitan Statistical Areas and a rural area covering much or all of a state. Such changes are subject to a budget neutrality requirement.

Premiums

All Medicare+Choice coordinated care plans, including HMOs, PSOs, and PPOs, must have submitted (by May 1998):

- adjusted community rate (ACR) proposals for basic and supplemental benefits;
- the plan's premium for the basic and supplemental benefits;
- a description of cost sharing and the actuarial value of cost sharing for basic and supplemental benefits; and
- a description of any additional benefits and the value of these benefits.

State Taxes

States can no longer tax the premium revenue of Medicare+Choice plans.

Health Care Prepayment Plans (HCPPs)

HCPPs are paid in a manner similar to cost plans, but only for part of the Medicare benefit package. HCPPs do not cover Medicare Part A services (inpatient hospital care, skilled nursing, hospice, and some home health care). However, some HCPPs arrange for services and can file Part A claims for their members.

Plan User Fees

Medicare+Choice plans and Section 1876 contractors must contribute their pro rata share, as determined by the DHHS, of estimated costs related to enrollment and dissemination of information, and certain counseling and assistance programs. The DHHS is authorized to collect user fees that are limited in the aggregate to:

- $200 million in fiscal year 1998;
- $150 million in fiscal year 1999;
- $100 million in fiscal year 2000 and beyond.

■ Quality Requirements

As the number of Medicare beneficiaries enrolled in managed care plans increases, HCFA works closely with states, insurers, health care professionals, and consumers to ensure quality of care. Medicare+Choice plans must undergo external quality reviews by independent review organizations. The DHHS is authorized to waive the external review requirement if the Medicare+Choice plan demonstrates a record of excellence in meeting quality assurance standards and complies with other applicable requirements. Plans are considered to have met internal quality assurance requirements if they are accredited by a private organization approved by the DHHS.

Beyond accreditation, several other quality initiatives are under way.

Medicare HEDIS

This HCFA effort with the Kaiser Family Foundation intends to establish a proven performance measurement system that minimizes the reporting burdens on managed care plans that serve Medicare beneficiaries. The new measures help plans improve the quality of their care and support efforts to improve the health status of beneficiaries.

Foundation for Accountability (FACCT)

This collaborative effort between private and public health care purchasers (including HCFA) and consumer groups develops outcome measures that compare the quality of care delivered in managed care settings to what is provided in fee-for-service settings. FACCT endorsed three condition-specific outcome measures—diabetes, depression, and breast cancer—that the RAND Corporation is testing for HCFA.

■ Reporting and Audit Requirements

In addition to reporting requirements cited above, Medicare+Choice plans must report:

Encounter Data

Effective January 1, 1998, the DHHS requires current Medicare managed care contractors to submit hospital encounter data that cover the period beginning July 1, 1997. On or after July 1, 1998, the DHHS is authorized to establish other encounter data reporting requirements for Medicare+Choice plans. This applies to current 1876 risk contractors that transition to the new program on January 1, 1999.

Fiscal Health

As a part of the monitoring and compliance process, Medicare+Choice plans must demonstrate fiscal soundness by disclosing financial information that includes data on business transactions involving property transfers and trades,

Table 7.2

Key Implementation Dates of the Medicare+Choice Program

Provision	Date
Enactment of the Balanced Budget Act of 1997, Public Law 105-33	August 5, 1997
Convening notice for negotiated rule-making to establish federal solvency standards for PSOs published in the *Federal Register*	September 19, 1997
Medicare+Choice plans begin reporting encounter data	January 1, 1998
Fiscal solvency standards for PSOs published in the *Federal Register*	April 1, 1998
Interim final register with contracting standards for Medicare+Choice plans published in the *Federal Register*	June 1, 1998
Special information campaign to inform eligible beneficiaries about Medicare+Choice options; 1876 risk plans must accept any new enrollees during the coordinated information campaign	November 1, 1998
1876 risk-based plans must transition to Medicare+Choice program	January 1, 1999
Elimination of HCPP option for entities eligible to contract as Medicare+Choice managed care plan	January 1, 1999
Termination of 1876 cost contracts	January 1, 2003

loans, and extensions of credit. Fiscal solvency standards for PSOs are to be established on a different track: a negotiated rule-making process, or through the DHHS if such a process is not successful.

HEDIS

As of January 1997, HCFA required plans to submit Medicare HEDIS data.

Annual Audit

The DHHS must annually audit the financial records of at least one-third of Medicare+Choice plans. The audit includes a review of data related to Medicare utilization, costs, and computation of the ACR. The audit process is monitored by the U.S. General Accounting Office.

■ Conclusion

Medicare managed care enrollment varies greatly depending on geographic location. Nationally, three-fourths of Medicare beneficiaries now have a choice of at least one managed care plan while more than half have a choice of two or more plans in their respective geographic areas. The majority of Medicare beneficiaries enrolled in managed care plans live in California, Florida, Oregon, New York, Arizona, and Hawaii.

With the new Medicare+Choice program, HCFA assumes the roles of purchaser and consumer protection agency, not just administrator of a government program. In its effort to offer more choice to Medicare beneficiaries, HCFA hopes to increase managed care enrollment and reduce the number of beneficiaries in its traditional fee-for-service programs (which have few cost containment features). By placing contracting health plan options "at risk" for government payments, HCFA can more accurately budget and can expand its emphasis on quality outcomes through additional reporting requirements.

Table 7.2 presents a summary of selected key dates related to the implementation of the Medicare+Choice program.

■ Key Terms

Adjusted average per
  capita cost (AAPCC)
"Age-ins"
Amount per member,
  per month
Annual audit
Balanced Budget Act of
  1997 (BBA '97)
Beneficiary eligibility
Competitive Medical
  Plan
Coordinated care plans
Disclosure rules

Encounter data
Enrollment,
  disenrollment
Foundation for
  Accountability
  (FACCT)
Health Care Prepayment
  Plan (HCPP)
Medical Savings Account
  (MSA)
Medicare+Choice
Payment rates

Plan user fees
Private fee-for-service
  plans
Provider participation
Public Law 105–33, the
  Balanced Budget Act
  of 1997 (BBA '97)
Quality requirements
Religious, fraternal
  benefit society plans
Section 1876 contracts
Special Information
  Campaign

Chapter 8

STATE GOVERNMENT AS A PURCHASER OF MANAGED CARE

■ Introduction

States purchase health care for two major population groups: state employees and Medicaid beneficiaries. Most states are also responsible for providing benefits to other groups (e.g., the homeless, mentally ill, and substance abusers). Like other major purchasers of health care, state governments seek ways to control costs, such as slowing the rate of cost increases. One promising cost containment method is the enrollment of state beneficiaries in managed care plans. During the past decade, governors, program managers, and state legislatures have embraced the managed care solution to achieve cost containment and ensure quality.

■ Medicaid Managed Care History

Medicaid's influence on managed care began in the 1970s. Initially, Medicaid beneficiary enrollment in managed care was voluntary. Those health plans that did enroll Medicaid providers were primarily located in states with a significant commercial managed care presence, such as Wisconsin, Minnesota, Washington, and California. In other states, Medicaid managed care enrollment became important in a few large cities: Detroit, Baltimore, and New York. In general, Medicaid managed care enrollment remained modest across the country.

The 1980s emphasis on managed care extended to Medicaid programs. A number of states—Colorado, Kansas, Kentucky, Michigan, Missouri, and Utah—began to operate primary health care provider model programs. In 1981 Congress enacted Section 1915(b) of the Social Security Act, authorizing the DHHS to grant special waivers permitting a state to limit provider choice and to mandate that Medicaid beneficiaries enroll either with a Primary Care Case Manager (PCCM) or in a managed care plan. In 1982, Arizona, operating under a Section 1115 waiver from the federal government, embarked on a statewide, all-at-risk managed care program. Only a few states took advantage of the new 1915(b) waivers (Missouri, Kansas, Pennsylvania, Wisconsin). By 1990 there had been little growth beyond 1980 levels in Medicaid managed care. (Note: In a PCCM program, the Medicaid beneficiary is assigned to a single primary health care provider (PCCM), who furnishes primary care and authorizes access to specialists. The care manager is paid a modest monthly case management fee—typically $3 to $5 per month—but all medical services are paid directly by the Medicaid program on a fee-for-service basis.)

Managed care enrollment in state Medicaid programs exploded in the 1990s. The growth was fueled by the public interest in national health care reform, increased penetration of managed care into the private sector, and the promise of cost containment. Cost containment is an important consideration for a program that had experienced dramatic growth in both number of beneficiaries and medical care inflation. The Medicaid program covers multiple low-income populations: single parents and their children (constituting the majority of managed care enrollees), pregnant women, disabled individuals, and the elderly. Evaluations from the Arizona program that demonstrated both cost containment and improvement in quality of care spurred more states to seek statewide health reform waivers under Section 1115. Oregon and Tennessee began statewide managed care Medicaid waiver programs in 1993; Hawaii and Rhode Island in 1994; and Delaware in 1996. Between 1992 and 1996, the total Medicaid population enrolled in some form of managed care increased from 11.75 to 40.10 percent (see Table 8.1). By June 30, 1996, a majority of the Medicaid managed care enrollees were in some type of at-risk plan.

■ The Medicaid Managed Care Picture Today

Enrollment Outlook

The popularity of managed care systems for Medicaid programs continues to grow. In late 1996 and 1997, several more states, including those with very large Medicaid populations (California, New York, Illinois, and Texas), obtained federal waivers to mandate enrollment in capitated plans. By mid-1998, managed care enrollment is predicted to exceed 1996 levels by at least three million individuals. Most of the enrollment growth is expected in plans and not in the PCCM system.

Table 8.1

Managed Care Trends

	Total Medicaid population	FFS population	Managed care population	Percent managed care enrollment
1991	28,280,000	25,583,603	2,696,397	9.53%
1992	30,926,390	27,291,874	3,634,516	11.75%
1993	33,430,051	28,621,100	4,808,951	14.39%
1994	33,634,000	25,839,750	7,794,250	23.17%
1995	33,373,000	23,573,000	9,800,000	29.37%
1996	33,241,147	19,911,028	13,330,119	40.10%

SOURCE: 1996 Medicaid Managed Care Enrollment Report, Office of Managed Care, Health Care Financing Administration, U.S. Department of Health and Human Services. Figures are as of June 30 of each year.

The Balanced Budget Act of 1997 relieved states of the obligation to seek a federal waiver to require beneficiaries to enroll in managed care plans or to be assigned to a primary care provider. Undoubtedly, this will further fuel the use of managed care systems by the states.

Diversity of Plans and Scope of Benefits

As used by Medicaid, "managed care" can mean a program as simple as the PCCM model described above or as comprehensive as enrolling beneficiaries into a fully capitated plan that provides all health care services.

The PCCM system is useful for controlling utilization of medical care and ensuring some coordination of the care of the beneficiary. Although PCCM systems are effective in ensuring continuity of care for the chronically ill, they offer neither the flexibility in benefit packages nor the predictability of cost found in at-risk capitated plans. The Medicaid program pays the managed care plan a fixed monthly amount and prescribes those benefits the plan must provide. A plan can, however, offer additional or atypical benefits (parenting classes, weight reduction clinics, etc.) at its own expense if it believes in the cost effectiveness of doing so.

The predominant Medicaid managed care model continues to be the general medical plan. Variations include:

■ full benefits in the general MCO contract;

■ limited benefits in the general MCO contract (prescription drugs, family planning services, and immunizations are sometimes "carved out" and left in the fee-for-service reimbursement system); and

99

■ a separate risk contract for specified benefits, such as behavioral health or substance abuse.

There are policy arguments for and against carve-outs and special purpose plans. On the plus side, they give individuals access to specialized providers who are experienced with the population or condition; on the negative side, they raise questions of accountability and coordination of care.

A few demonstration projects now target special segments of the Medicaid population. For example, the District of Columbia contracts with a plan to cover services for handicapped children; Massachusetts initiated a shared-risk plan to serve a small number of Medicaid beneficiaries with very complicated, multiple medical conditions.

Most states do not enroll persons covered by both Medicaid and Medicare—the "dual-eligibles"—in managed care plans. Long-term care services are customarily reimbursed on a fee-for-service basis. Minnesota is experimenting with a managed care structure that combines Medicaid and Medicare coverage to serve the dual-eligible population. Colorado, Massachusetts, and Maine are seeking federal approval for similar demonstrations.

Purchasing for Value

As a state's experience with managed care grows, the attitudes of program managers change. Managers begin to refer to their state's role as "purchaser," rather than as "insurer," and use their vast purchasing power to influence the quality of medical care. To do so, a variety of "tools" are used, including:

Data Sets

Initially, New York and Massachusetts adopted some of the HEDIS 2.5 (*Health Plan Employer Data and Information Set*) measures for evaluating the quality of a plan's performance for its Medicaid clients. However, HEDIS was deemed inadequate to measure care for a population that comprised primarily low-income women and children. In response to the need, the National Committee for Quality Assurance (NCQA) published a special Medicaid HEDIS data set in February 1996.

The second edition of HEDIS (HEDIS 3.0), published in January 1997, incorporates most of the Medicaid HEDIS material and creates a single data set applicable to both commercial and Medicaid populations. A 1996 survey conducted by the American Public Welfare Association and NCQA found that 31 of the 38 Medicaid programs that contract with MCOs use some or all of these measures, and over 70 percent expect to have some data by the end of 1997.

States also use encounter (utilization) data and financial reports to monitor the care given to their beneficiaries and to ensure a plan's continued fiscal health.

External Reviews

Organizations external to both the state government and the plans are used to monitor performance. These include accreditation reviews by JCAHO or by NCQA, and program audits by agencies such as peer review organizations (PROs). The Balanced Budget Act of 1997 requires the Department of Health and Human Services, in consultation with the states, to develop protocols for external reviews of Medicaid participating plans.

Consumer Satisfaction Surveys

Monitoring consumer satisfaction with the Medicaid population poses a unique challenge. Testing of various approaches to survey Medicaid beneficiaries is under way in an attempt to overcome obstacles such as language barriers, lack of telephones, or cultural biases. Some techniques employed to evaluate and enhance consumer satisfaction include hot lines with 800 numbers, ombudsman programs, and consumer advocacy groups to assist Medicaid beneficiaries who encounter problems with a plan.

Quality Improvement Studies

Participating plans are required to conduct one or more studies each year to measure their own performance in a particular area, and then devise, implement, and evaluate interventions to improve it. For example, a plan might determine that the incidence of low birthweight babies is higher than expected and develop special activities for pregnant enrollees. The before-and-after data, plus a description of the intervention, constitutes a quality improvement study for a plan. The studies are sent to the state and used as technical assistance for other plans.

Incentives and Sanctions

States employ a variety of incentives and sanctions in their quality improvement activities. Plans rated as high quality may be rewarded with a larger share of the "auto enrollments" (beneficiaries who do not select a plan and are assigned by the state). Another incentive is public recognition, which can result from the publication of results of consumer surveys or quality assessments in the newspaper, or by highlighting a plan's successful quality improvement efforts in a brochure.

Sanctions are imposed for poor performance and may include restricted enroll-ment pending remedial action, imposing temporary management on a plan, allowing beneficiaries to disenroll immediately, and, ultimately, termination or non-renewal of the health plan's contract.

■ Special State Policy Considerations

Protecting the Traditional Care Provider

Traditionally, a special set of providers (often referred to as the "safety net") serves the Medicaid and medically indigent populations in a given area. These providers include:

- public hospitals and university medical centers;
- children's hospitals;
- neighborhood health centers;
- rural health centers; and
- clinics serving the homeless, migrant worker families, and persons with AIDS.

A growing managed care enrollment creates a real fear in the affected commu-nity that these providers may stop receiving Medicaid patients or be inade-quately reimbursed for Medicaid services. It is in the community's interest to maintain the availability of these resources. The challenge today is to achieve an appropriate balance between the state's role as a prudent purchaser and the state's desire to support the continued availability of these vital providers. To address this issue, Colorado, Rhode Island, and Massachusetts encourage their public hospitals and clinic networks to form a managed care plan with which the state then contracts directly.

Establishing a Fair Rate Structure

Managed care plans regularly urge purchasers to "risk adjust" capitation rates to address differences between enrollee populations. States usually have a number of rates, reflecting differences in age, sex, and, sometimes, the region of the state in which the beneficiary lives. In 1997, Colorado and Maryland launched interesting new Medicaid rate adjustment demonstrations. Both states attempt to capture the differences in resources used by enrollees with different condi-tions (e.g., sickle cell anemia, AIDS, or diabetes). These demonstrations are be-ing carefully watched by the managed care industry.

Minimizing the Burden of Compliance

Managing a managed care plan in today's environment is not easy. The quality assurance demands, new federal and state laws, and a rapidly changing fiscal environment (as plans merge and providers change) put pressure on a plan's leadership. New requirements, especially in quality assurance, present a significant compliance burden for smaller plans that lack the resources to buy sophisticated computer systems or management assistance. When a state establishes consistent expectations, particularly in reporting/data elements and formats for Medicare, Medicaid, and commercial purchasers, it significantly reduces the compliance burden on a plan and increases the opportunities for comparative analysis and evaluation.

To that end, Minnesota and Massachusetts developed their Medicaid contract specifications in concert with other state programs. In Minnesota, the state employee program and the Medicaid program contracts are almost identical. In Massachusetts, the Medicaid program and the mental health department have a formal agreement: Medicaid purchases services for both and they jointly develop the performance standards.

■ Conclusion

By 1998, managed care systems, especially fully-at-risk managed care plans, have become a major element in the provider community that serves state programs. State program managers are aggressive, quality-oriented purchasers of care, not passive bill-payers. As managed care evolves, new business opportunities emerge for both purchasers and providers. The strong emphasis on preventive, primary, and multidisciplinary care encourages new provider groupings and patient management techniques. The drive for accountability spawns new measurement tools and research. These factors increase the likelihood that states will continue to be able to purchase high-quality benefits from MCOs for their citizens.

■ Key Terms

"Auto enrollments"
Consumer satisfaction
  surveys
"Dual-eligibles"
External reviews
Incentives and sanctions

Joint Commission on
  Accreditation of
  Healthcare
  Organizations
  (JCAHO)
Medicaid HEDIS data set

National Committee for
  Quality Assurance
  (NCQA)
Peer Review
  Organizations
  (PROs)

Primary care case
   manager (PCCM)
Purchasing for value

Quality improvement
   studies
"Safety net"

Section 1115 waiver
Section 1915(b) of the
   Social Security Act

Section III

THE INS AND OUTS OF "CARVE-OUTS"

This section describes those health services that are not included in capitated benefits and are reimbursed separately on a predetermined fee-for-service basis. MCOs may manage these services directly or through subcontractors. This section addresses four common services: pharmacy benefits, dental care, behavioral health care, and vision care. Each chapter addresses the unique features of a service, how it adapts to managed care, and specific issues that facilitate or hinder the success of managed care.

Chapter 9 covers the pharmaceutical programs that are an essential component of medical benefits coverage but because of tremendous increases in the cost of drugs and their wide use are often managed under separate programs. Chapter 10 describes dental managed care programs and their differences from medical managed care. Chapter 11 discusses the issues that arise in the application of managed care to mental health services, in part because of the training and traditional work styles that pervade behavioral health services. Chapter 12 addresses the application of managed care to visual health services.

Chapter 9

PHARMACY BENEFIT MANAGEMENT PROGRAMS

■ Introduction

Prescription drug benefit management has evolved tremendously since the late 1980s, away from the minor drug programs that once were a plan "throw-in," with minimal charge to the employer and minimal copayment ($1-$3 per prescription). These programs received little attention until the 1980s, when double-digit price increases by manufacturers and new drug products to treat diseases such as ulcers (which were previously difficult to cure) caused insurers to consider new ways to manage the cost of prescription drug benefits. During this same time, biotechnology also emerged, resulting in drug therapies that cost in excess of $1,000 per prescription.

■ Program Growth

Beginning in the 1960s and continuing into the early 1980s, pharmacy benefit management consisted primarily of contracting with pharmacy networks to develop a basis for prescription reimbursement and claims processing. Even into the late 1980s, prescriptions were processed using "home-grown" paper claim forms, until the adoption of the Universal Claim Form (UCF) created the standard for the electronic submission of prescription drug claims. Most often, claim forms were batched by a pharmacy and sent to the claims processor for payment. A health plan or payer realized savings from network discounts (instead of reimbursement based on "usual and customary" charges) and through cost-effective claims processing. An administrative fee paid to claim processor services typically is 50 percent less than in-house processing costs.

Today, prescription drug programs command center stage. Faced with an escalating cost trend, most health plans created internal departments or contracted with pharmacy benefit management companies (PBMs) that employ many tactics to improve the quality and the financial outlook of their prescription drug benefit programs. Today's programs:

- process claims online, in real time, while the patient is in the pharmacy;
- perform complete claims adjudication in several seconds, even with extensive claim edits; and
- employ clinical edits to help prevent dispensing of potentially harmful or inappropriate drugs.

MCOs are creating more sophisticated and complex benefit designs to halt the upward trend of drug costs. They employ clinical management programs that are designed to improve patient care and control cost, such as:

- formularies, or lists of approved drugs for use by physicians;
- therapeutic/generic product switch programs;
- drug utilization review programs to detect inappropriate drug use; and
- disease management programs.

■ Key Components of a Pharmacy Benefit Management Program

The following are the components of a pharmacy benefit management program and represent a variety of tactics that a health plan can implement to achieve pharmacy program goals.

Pharmacy Networks

"The larger the pharmacy network the better" was the initial view of most purchasers of prescription drug benefits. Many purchasers even specified distance criteria for pharmacies (e.g., one participating pharmacy within five miles of each employee's home). Given the favorable reimbursement rates early on, most pharmacies readily agreed to participate in networks.

The national expansion of managed care programs reduced the reimbursement rates for pharmacies and resulted in smaller networks. A restricted network

Table 9.1

Two Pharmacy Network Designs and Associated Reimbursement Rates

Network	Participating pharmacies	AWP	Dispensing fee	Possible incentives
1	80 to 90 percent	10 to 13 percent	$2.50 to $4	$0.50 to $ 1 per generic prescription
2	50 percent	13 to 16 percent	$1.50 to $3	$0.50 to $10 per qualifying prescription

SOURCE: *WellPoint* Pharmacy Management.

approach continues to gain popularity, as MCOs seek additional methods to reduce cost increases. Under this approach, MCOs first contract with major pharmacy chains to anchor the network and then contract with strategically located, independent pharmacies to complete it. That approach allows less (but still adequate) access for members compared with a wider network. In exchange for possible increases in members' travel, purchasers realize lower prescription drug program costs and member cost-sharing is more stable.

Pharmacy reimbursement is usually structured as a discount from the drug's average wholesale price (AWP) set by the manufacturer, plus a professional or dispensing fee. In the 1970s, reimbursement was often set at 100 percent AWP, or even AWP plus a percentage. In today's networks, discounts range from AWP minus 10 to 20 percent. Dispensing fees of $3.50-$5 in the past are now $1-$4 less depending on network size and geographic location. Pharmacies may receive incentives to dispense generic, formulary, or preferred-formulary drugs. Several national PBMs developed a "Pay for Performance" program to reward pharmacies for meeting or exceeding program goals and objectives. Table 9.1 illustrates two network designs and associated reimbursement rates.

Claim Processing

In the late 1960s and early 1970s, pharmacy claims were processed when a member submitted a paper claim and a pharmacy receipt. These claims were processed by the health plan in conjunction with a major medical benefit. The member was reimbursed a percentage of the billed charges after a program deductible was satisfied. The next generation of pharmacy processing (pharmacy card programs) required the participating pharmacy to submit a paper claim form on behalf of the member. The member made a copayment of up to $3.

Table 9.2

Clinical and Administrative Edits Used in Electronic Claim Processing

Administrative	Clinical
■ eligibility checking	■ early refill
■ duplicate claim checking	■ duplicate therapy
■ copay determination	■ drug-drug interactions
■ benefit limits checking	■ drug-disease conflicts
■ benefit maximum	■ drug-age conflicts
■ in-network vs. out-of-network benefits	■ drug-gender conflicts
■ exclusions	■ minimum dose
■ day's supply limitation	■ maximum dose
■ quantity limitations	■ drug-pregnancy warnings
■ high cost limits	■ pediatric precautions
■ deductible payments	■ geriatric precautions
■ coordination of benefits	■ late refill alert
■ network pricing	

The prescription drug rider was almost a giveaway to employers because of the low cost of prescription drugs.

Pharmacy-submitted claims quickly became standardized with adoption of the Universal Claim Form. Pharmacy claim processors keyed claims manually and paid the pharmacies on behalf of the carrier. Administrative fees ranged from $.50–$1.50 per claim. Batch processing brought efficiency as the cost to process batch claims fell below the cost of a total manual effort.

The electronic submission of the prescription information directly from the pharmacy to the claim processor introduced the next generation of pharmacy claim processing in the late 1980s. The technology evolved to become online, real-time claim submission and adjudication that allows eligibility and benefit checking at the point of service (see Table 9.2). This process eliminates "good faith" payments to a pharmacy (i.e., one-time payments made in the event a pharmacy renders services to an ineligible member).

Administrative Fees

Well into the 1990s, the administrative fees for prescription claim processing continued to erode, to the point that it is now common to find fees in the mid-$0.20 per claim range for high-volume carriers or health plans. Standards for

Table 9.3

Processing Performance Standards

Processing	3 seconds or less
	95 percent of the time
System Availability	24 hours a day/7 days a week
	99 percent of the time

performance are common (see Table 9.3). Today claim processing is considered a commodity. However, flexibility and customization in processing are critical for health plans that are innovative and competitive.

Benefit Design

Since the 1960s, dramatic changes have occurred in prescription drug benefit designs, including the practice of covering most drugs (except drugs to treat obesity, vitamins, and over-the-counter [OTC] products) and not limiting the days' supply of medications. With the advent of high technology and biotechnology, today's benefit programs exclude drugs that are not essential or medically necessary for all patients. Benefit designs are now very complex, as can be seen in Table 9.4.

Table 9.4

Typical Pharmaceutical Benefit Designs

Copayments	Common exclusions	Benefit limitations

■ Fixed copays: $5 to $25
■ Percent copays: 10 percent to 50 percent
■ Tiered copays:
  ■ $5 for generics/$10 to $20 for brands
  ■ $5 for generics/$10 to $15 for formulary brands/$20 to $25 for non-formulary brands
  ■ $5 to $10 for formulary drugs/$15 to $25 for non-formulary drugs
	■ Drugs for cosmetic use (Rogaine, Retin-A)
	■ OTC products (except insulin)
	■ Appetite suppressants
	■ Injectable drugs (except self-injectable)
	■ Human growth hormone
	■ Fertility drugs
	■ Contraceptives (oral and devices)
	■ Investigational and experimental drugs
	■ Non-formulary drugs (for plans with closed formularies)
	■ Nicotine replacement therapy
		■ Retail days' supply (typically 34 days or 100 units)
		■ Mail service days' supply (60 to 90 days)
		■ Nicotine replacement therapy limited to one course of treatment per year or lifetime
		■ Maximum of X tablets per prescription or per months of therapy (e.g., Viagra)

111

Table 9.5

Comparison of Retail and Mail Service Fees

Criteria	Retail	Mail Service
AWP discount	13 percent	18 percent
Dispensing fee	$3	$1
Days' supply	30	90
AWP cost of medication ($1.00/tablet)	$30	$90
Discounted cost of medication	$26.10	$73.80
Copayment*	$5	$5
Overall cost for 90 days	$72.30	$69.80 (3.5 percent savings)

*If the retail and mail service copay was $10, then the retail option would provide an 11.6 percent savings over mail service.

Mail Service Programs

Mail service pharmacies have grown tremendously since the mid-1980s, and now account for more than 10 percent of all prescriptions filled annually. These programs gained popularity because of the aggressive discounts offered by mail service pharmacies and the convenience of home delivery for members.

Mail service programs usually provide a 90-day supply of medication for a single copay and a single dispensing fee. While such an arrangement was attractive several years ago, today it warrants a second look. With retail reimbursement eroding significantly, an MCO must carefully consider the discounts, dispensing fees, and copays when developing a mail service benefit. At times, the savings on discount and dispensing fees may not make up for the loss of copayments (see Table 9.5).

Mail service pharmacies also emerged as successful operators of formulary or therapeutic-switching programs. Without a member waiting for a prescription, the mail service pharmacist can contact (usually within a day) the prescribing physician to request a medication change that results in savings for the MCO. A mail service pharmacy may gain additional revenue from pharmaceutical man-ufacturers that realize an increase in sales of their drugs.[48] In most cases, both the physician and patient must agree to the change before it is finalized.

Mail service pharmacies are highly automated and provide an accurate, conve-nient service for patients. In the future, these pharmacies will be challenged to continue to reduce operating costs, improve delivery turnaround to patients, and provide additional services related to the total care management of the patient.

Customer Service

An MCO's pharmacy service program is essential in today's claim processing environment. Pharmacies rely on the MCO's service representatives to answer questions about a member's eligibility, benefits, claim reimbursement, copay, and other benefit restrictions. The representative can literally observe a claim submission to ensure the accurate transmission of every data element. The service generally operates with a toll-free phone number and is available 12 hours per weekday and eight hours on weekends and holidays. The service is expected to operate efficiently and meet precise performance standards, such as:

- speed of answering: < 20 seconds
- wait time: < 20 seconds
- abandon rate: < 5 percent
- satisfied callers: > 90 percent

■ Clinical Quality Programs

MCOs rely on clinical management programs, such as a drug formulary and utilization review, to improve program quality and to lower costs. These programs are often established and overseen by a pharmacy and therapeutic (P&T) committee operated by the health plan. The mission of a P&T committee is to ensure that included in the pharmaceuticals in the prescription drug formulary are the most appropriate, rational, and affordable products for use. The committee recommends guidelines for appropriate use of medications and develops policies regarding the evaluation, selection, and therapeutic use of pharmaceuticals. The committee creates value for both providers and patients by developing and maintaining a select list of products, which benefits both patient care and program costs. A P&T committee typically comprises physicians, pharmacists, and other health care personnel as voting members. Physician specialists attend when their particular area of expertise is discussed. Meetings are usually held quarterly. The committee must be organized and operated in a manner to ensure its objectivity and enhance its credibility.

Drug Formulary

A drug formulary is a list of drugs, approved by a panel of health care practitioners, that serves to guide prescribers to select the most appropriate drug for a given patient. The list's purpose is to promote rational, cost-effective drug

---

Sample Formulary

Anti-Infective Agents (Oral)

Anthelmintes

$ Mebendazole (generic Vermox)

$$ Thiabendazole (Mintezol)

Antibiotics

Cephalosporins

$ Cephalexin (generic Keflex)

$$ Cefaclor (generic Ceclor)

$$$ Cefadroxie (generic Duricef)

$$$$ Cefixime (Suprax)

$$$$ Cefpodoxime Proxetil (Vantin)

$$$$ Cefprozil (Cefzil)

$$$$$ Cefuroxime (Ceftin)

Cost Key					
$	=	<$10	$$$$	=	$40-$60
$$	=	$10-$20	$$$$$	=	$60-$80
$$$	=	$20-$40	$$$$$$	=	>$80

Figure 9.1

SOURCE: WellPoint Pharmacy Management.

therapy (see Figure 9.1). As a dynamic document—constantly reviewed and updated by a committee of experts—it is an effective way to keep health care professionals up-to-date with all the new drugs on the market. Health plans print a formulary and distribute it to all physicians and pharmacies participating in the network. A formulary may include:

■ a drug list by therapeutic class and by generic and brand name within each class;

■ any preferred drugs;

■ a relative price index that tells the prescriber the cost of each product or therapy to the health plan;

■ policies and procedures;

■ treatment guidelines; and

■ outcome studies and disease management information.

114

Drugs selected for formulary inclusion are evaluated on the following criteria:

- efficacy/effectiveness (relative to other therapies);
- safety (side effects or drug interactions);
- pharmacokinetic advantages (dosing/compliance);
- product uniqueness (clinical alternatives);
- cost of therapy; and
- outcomes.

There are three basic types of drug formularies.

Open Formulary: a comprehensive list of drugs with few, if any, restrictions or limitations. An open formulary primarily serves as a reference document for the prescriber. Typically, there is no financial impact on the member/patient when a physician prescribes a non-formulary agent.

Closed Formulary: a limited list of approved drugs. Closed formularies, often associated with institutions and strongly managed HMOs, are gaining momentum among health plans today. A closed formulary promotes rational prescribing and provides cost savings through the appropriate use of generics and first-line brand products. In a closed formulary, a non-formulary drug may be rejected as a benefit or require a prior authorization (a process for approving non-formulary drugs) to ensure that the drug is medically necessary and appropriately prescribed. The patient may not receive the prescribed drug. The closed formulary option typically provides the health plan with pharmacy cost savings. However, customer satisfaction suffers when sufficient educational information is not distributed to the member, prescriber, and pharmacist. Closed formularies save MCOs 5–15 percent of program costs, depending on how limited the formulary is and the degree of health plan clinical management. Variations are:

- Positive formulary: a list of those drugs approved for use by an MCO. This formulary example lists drugs that are included in the benefit.
- Negative formulary: a list of drugs that are not approved for use by an MCO. This formulary example lists drugs that are not included in the benefit.

Restricted Formulary: a hybrid that is not as restricted as the closed formulary but lists fewer drugs than an open formulary. This type of formulary provides some cost management opportunities, most likely in the top 10–15 therapeutic classes.

Therapeutic Interchange

Therapeutic interchange occurs when an originally prescribed drug is replaced by one that is equivalent in terms of effectiveness and results.[49] Therapeutic interchange can only occur after the prescriber approves such a change. Before doing so, a panel of physicians must have determined in advance that the patient will experience the same outcome with either drug. While the goal is to improve the outcome of medical care to the patient, the process does not always result in a lower drug cost. A recommendation may stipulate, for example, that a patient receive a once-a-day dose, rather than a three-times-a-day dose. In that case, the cost of the prescription may be higher. However, the patient's medication compliance (and thus his or her overall care) should improve. Therapeutic interchanges are commonly used by MCOs today, but they have occurred in other settings (hospitals, nursing homes) for many years. A tool to help better manage a prescription drug program, therapeutic interchange is designed to improve care and overall cost savings.

Pharmaceutical Manufacturer Discounts/Rebates

Pharmaceutical manufacturers commonly provide discounts or rebates to MCOs for purchases of the manufacturer's products that are made by the MCO's enrollees. These discounts are based on compliance with requirements that usually include listing the drug on the health plan's formulary, covering the drug under the patient's prescription drug program, and the actual use of the products. Rebates can provide savings of 2–5 percent of the total drug expenditure. The more a particular product is utilized relative to its competition, the higher may be the rebate or discount.

Treatment Guidelines

Treatment guidelines provide objective, unbiased criteria so that prescribers have up-to-date information on therapeutically appropriate and cost-effective drug therapy. The treatment guidelines are based on a review of the medical literature, on community medical standards, and on a review of the policies and recommendations of respected national health and medical organizations. Treatment guidelines are incorporated into disease and therapy management programs. Since treatment guidelines are based on actual outcomes, they are more acceptable to physicians and improve the prescribing of medications (see Figure 9.2).

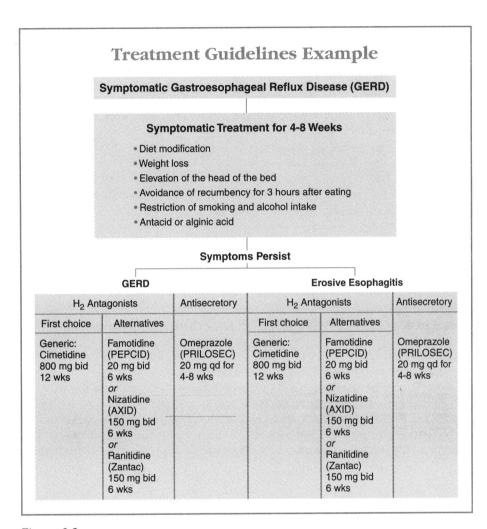

Treatment Guidelines Example

Symptomatic Gastroesophageal Reflux Disease (GERD)

Symptomatic Treatment for 4-8 Weeks

- Diet modification
- Weight loss
- Elevation of the head of the bed
- Avoidance of recumbency for 3 hours after eating
- Restriction of smoking and alcohol intake
- Antacid or alginic acid

Symptoms Persist

GERD			Erosive Esophagitis		
H₂ Antagonists		Antisecretory	H₂ Antagonists		Antisecretory
First choice	Alternatives		First choice	Alternatives	
Generic: Cimetidine 800 mg bid 12 wks	Famotidine (PEPCID) 20 mg bid 6 wks *or* Nizatidine (AXID) 150 mg bid 6 wks *or* Ranitidine (Zantac) 150 mg bid 6 wks	Omeprazole (PRILOSEC) 20 mg qd for 4-8 wks	Generic: Cimetidine 800 mg bid 12 wks	Famotidine (PEPCID) 20 mg bid 6 wks *or* Nizatidine (AXID) 150 mg bid 6 wks *or* Ranitidine (Zantac) 150 mg bid 6 wks	Omeprazole (PRILOSEC) 20 mg qd for 4-8 wks

Figure 9.2

SOURCE: WellPoint Pharmacy Management.

Prior Authorization

Prior authorization is a clinical process that allows health care professionals to review drug therapy and the patient's drug profile and determine the appropriateness of requested therapy. Designated for prior authorization are those drugs:

- with high potential for adverse reactions;
- that are frequently prescribed inappropriately;
- have high abuse potential; or
- that are second-line agents frequently prescribed as first-line.

When a drug is flagged for prior authorization, the prescribing physician is asked a series of questions and, if the established criteria are met, the prescription is approved. The process helps minimize patient inconvenience and dissatisfaction. For the MCO, prior authorization leads to appropriate drug use, which translates into more cost-effective outcomes.

Drug Utilization Review (DUR)

Drug utilization review (DUR) or drug use evaluation (DUE) encompasses the review of physician prescribing, pharmacist dispensing, and patients' use of drugs.[50] The goal of this program is to ensure high quality of service to the patient at an affordable cost through appropriate prescribing and use of drugs. DUR/DUE involves the following steps:

1. Develop modules and criteria to identify inappropriate use of medications.
2. Conduct data pulls to identify inappropriate use.
3. Compare the actual use to the criteria developed.
4. Prepare a clinical intervention with the prescriber, pharmacist, or patient.
5. Measure the results of the intervention.

There are three types of DUR/DUE programs: prospective, concurrent, and retrospective. Definitions vary according to the health care setting or one's perspective.

Prospective DUR

This form of DUR/DUE requires an action or intervention by a health care professional before the patient takes the medication. The prescriber may review educational materials from the health plan's clinical pharmacist regarding the appropriate use of certain medications. If the prescriber understands and agrees to the message and guidelines, then the next time a patient presents with the same disease or condition, the recommended medication is prescribed. Technology enables the prescriber to receive real-time information, via computer, regarding the patient's drug profile and guidelines for the use of particular medications. In this way, the prescriber either avoids writing a prescription for an inappropriate drug or changes the prescription before the patient receives the medication. Although the technology exists today, the integration of this process into the prescriber's daily routine is not yet fully accepted.

Concurrent DUR

This form of DUR/DUE relates to monitoring a patient on drug therapy and primarily occurs in a research setting, but it can also occur at the pharmacy. For example, a patient takes a medication prescribed by a specialist for the treatment of coronary artery disease. Then, the patient suffers a severe headache and presents at an urgent care center. The attending physician may prescribe a drug that conflicts with the current therapy if the patient fails to inform the physician about the prior medication. When a new prescription is entered into the pharmacy's online claim processing system, the drug-drug interaction is discovered. The pharmacist contacts the prescribing physician to change the medication to one appropriate for the patient.

Retrospective DUR

This form of DUR/DUE involves a review of the prescribing patterns of physicians, dispensing patterns of pharmacists, and drug use by patients on an after-the-fact basis.

- A prescriber-focused program analyzes the prescribing patterns of physicians regarding the use of formulary agents, generic drugs, length of therapy, and dosing of medications. Often, an individual prescriber is compared with peers in his or her specialty area or in the provider network or with best practice, as defined by the health plan.

- Pharmacy reviews compare the individual pharmacy to the entire pharmacy network for key performance indicators. In both situations, specific patient information is sent to either the prescriber or pharmacist for review.

- Patient drug profiles are reviewed over a period of time (usually three to six months) to identify inappropriate drug use, such as the overuse of controlled substances. The reviewer defines overuse/misuse/abuse of specific medications, and patients are identified for review. Next, the reviewer rules out patients on chronic pain therapy, such as cancer treatment, and develops a communication for the prescribing physician(s). A communication may be sent to the pharmacist(s) and to the patient. The goal is to correct the use of these drugs and place the patient on the most appropriate therapy.

Disease Management Programs

Disease management is defined many different ways. It is most commonly portrayed as an effort to reduce total health care expenditures through a coordi-

119

nated effort among health care professionals in regard to a particular disease state.[51] Each program incorporates many components, including:

■ patient education (medication compliance);

■ provider education: guidelines for treatment of the disease;

■ data analysis: integration of medical and pharmacy (lab data, if available);

■ cognitive services: reimbursing providers for additional training and patient counseling; and

■ case management services.

Disease management programs require an extensive data analysis of hospitalizations, emergency room visits, physician office visits, lab data, and prescription drug data associated with a specific diagnosis. The disease states frequently addressed today are:

■ asthma,

■ peptic ulcer disease,

■ diabetes,

■ depression,

■ congestive heart failure, and

■ hypertension.

For example, asthmatics are identified by using the asthma-specific ICD9 code and noting the presence of asthma-related drugs. Once patients are identified, they are stratified by severity of illness as determined by co-morbidities, extensive drug use, and frequency of resource utilization. The results assign patients into three categories:

■ high risk: intensive interventions;

■ medium risk: moderate interventions; or

■ low risk: educational program.

Depending on the severity of illness, a comprehensive approach is often required to significantly improve the situation. For high-risk-category patients, a recommended intensive approach includes patient educational materials, physician interventions, pharmacist counseling, and case management. A case manager may call to the patient to assess his or her quality of life and satisfaction with the program. Additionally, a demand management opportunity exists for patients to contact the case manager or educator with questions regarding their disease or therapy.

Outcomes are measured every quarter to every six months after the program is implemented. The outcome is expected to show significant improvement in the overall quality of care, which usually leads to an improvement in total health care cost for the enrollees.

Many companies that offer disease management programs only provide the educational component. With disease management emerging as one approach to controlling health care costs, it is important to determine if all the necessary components are present to achieve the overall goal.

Educational Programs

Programs designed to improve the prescribing and dispensing of medications are widely used by MCOs and their subcontractors. These programs fall into three categories:

1. Prescriber education: informs physicians and other prescribers of preferred medications on the formulary and offers information, including treatment guidelines, to improve the prescribing of medications.
2. Pharmacist training programs: enhance patient counseling skills for medication compliance and for specific disease management programs.
3. Patient educational information: informs patients about their disease and how to recognize warning signs; the importance of medication compliance; generic drugs; and questions to ask their doctor or pharmacist.

■ Pharmacy Program Reporting and Analysis

Timely and accurate program reporting is essential to today's pharmacy benefit manager. Pharmacy benefit plan reporting is usually available online, on-demand. Systems that incorporate Sybase or Oracle database software rapidly produce almost unlimited data cuts or sorts. This flexibility allows the benefit manager to make timely decisions and assists in case management.

Key indicators are monitored frequently to discover any unexpected trends. Most pharmacy program managers continuously review the following indicators:

■ average cost/prescription;

■ number of prescriptions per member;

■ generic use rate;

■ formulary use rate;

121

Table 9.6

Types of Drugs and Average Cost per Prescription

Type of drug	Average cost per prescription
Single-source brands	$40
Multi-source brands	$27
Generics	$8
Overall	$35

■ total cost per member; and

■ average copay per prescription.

These indicators help identify trends in cost and utilization and trigger actions by the manager to research certain aspects of the program. For instance, if the average cost per prescription increases significantly, is it because of manufacturer price increases? An increased use of brand drugs instead of generics? More expensive brand drugs? The drug mix is very important information to monitor, as Table 9.6 illustrates.

■ The greater the use of single-source brands, the less the opportunity to dispense cost-effective generics, increasing the average cost dramatically.

■ Cost is the reason many prescription drug programs designate a higher co-pay or member cost-sharing for a brand prescription.

Table 9.6 demonstrates the cost effectiveness of generic drugs. For every percentage point increase in the generic drug usage rate, total program costs are reduced by 0.4 to 0.7 percent.

Provider Profiling

Reports are generated to measure provider performance in the selection of the most cost-effective therapies. Prescribers are reviewed for individual performance and compared within a specialty with the health plan's determination of best practice or with the overall network performance. Prescriber profiles may adjust for patient mix to equalize the comparison. Providers that fall below expectations are contacted and, through a review process, opportunities for performance improvement are identified. Such opportunities may involve prescribing more formulary products or generic drugs.

Example of Provider Profiling

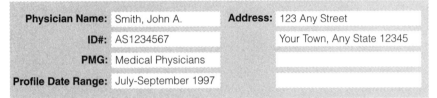

Physician Name:	Smith, John A.	**Address:**	123 Any Street
ID#:	AS1234567		Your Town, Any State 12345
PMG:	Medical Physicians		
Profile Date Range:	July-September 1997		

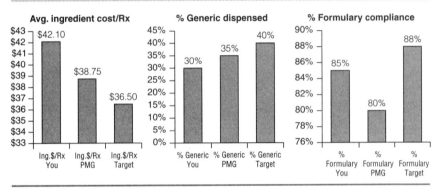

The Table below is a list of your most commonly prescribed drugs that have a cost-effective formulary alternative available.

Please review the information and contact your pharmacist with any questions you may have regarding your utilization.

Prescribed drug	Total Rxs	Average cost per Rx	Formulary alternative(s)	Average cost per alternative Rx	Potential cost savings
Voltaren XR	6	$64.21	Diclofenac, Ibuprofen, Naproxen	$34.36	$179.10
Glucotrol	5	$43.04	Glipizide, Glucotrol XL	$8.50	$172.70
Provera	3	$24.63	Medroxyprogesterone	$13.47	$33.48
Zocor	3	$93.43	Pravachol, Lescol, Lipitor	$80.18	$39.75
Zantac	3	$87.28	Ranitidine	$75.34	$35.82
Lopressor	2	$52.54	Metaprolol	$8.10	$88.88
Vaseretic	2	$104.81	Zestoretic	$53.68	$102.26
Dyazide	2	$36.31	Triamterene/HCTZ	$8.81	$55.00
Hismanal	2	$52.72	Allegra, Claritin, Zyrtec	$49.11	$7.22

Figure 9.3

SOURCE: WellPoint Pharmacy Management.

Patient Profiling

Important reports help determine when patients are taking multiple therapies that conflict with each other or that are inappropriate or unnecessary. Medication compliance, critical to therapy success, can be closely monitored for certain therapies. Typically, refill frequency and days of continuous therapy are measured. When a patient is found chronically noncompliant, the prescriber, pharmacist, and patient may be contacted, made aware of the situation, and actions are taken to improve compliance. The overall goal for patient monitoring is to improve the outcome of a particular therapy and to ensure appropriate medication use.

Drug Utilization

Reports by cost or number of prescriptions allow monitoring of therapeutic classes and top drugs. These reports track high-cost, high-tech products to ensure that prescribing complies with guidelines and that the drugs are not arbitrarily overutilized.

Disease Management and Outcomes

Outcomes are a significant component of disease management programs. A complete analysis of a year's data is conducted to determine the benefit to both the patient and the health plan. All cost, quality of life, and satisfaction factors are measured to establish a baseline, which is then compared with post-intervention results. Improvements are evaluated by:

- Economic outcomes: determine the cost of services provided for a particular disease state (e.g., cost of hospitalization, office visits, emergency room visits, labs, medications).

- Clinical outcomes: determine improvement in the care of the patient (e.g., higher degree of compliance to national guidelines for the treatment of asthma).

- Humanistic outcomes: determine the improvement in the patient's quality of life.

NCQA/HEDIS Reporting

MCOs seeking accreditation from the National Commission for Quality Assurance (NCQA) must comply with standards for pharmacy follow-up reporting and provide data for the pharmacy-specific indicators found in HEDIS 3.0. The effectiveness of care measurements include:

- Treating child's ear infection
- Cholesterol management of patients
- Beta-blocker treatment after heart attack
- Controlling high blood pressure
- Aspirin treatment after heart attack
- Prescription of antibiotics for prevention of HIV-related pneumonia
- Use of appropriate medications for people with asthma
- Screening for chemical dependency
- Monitoring of diabetes patients
- Continuation of depression treatment
- Availability of medication for patients with schizophrenia
- Appropriate use of psychotherapeutic medications

Pharmacy Benefit Management Companies (PBMs)

PBMs began primarily as claims processors in the 1960s, when employer groups, health insurance carriers, and other third-party administrators sought to improve the administrative costs of their pharmacy programs. In the 1980s, the term "PBM" emerged as health plans expected these organizations to provide more services to control the sharply rising costs of prescription drug benefits. Drug formularies, rebates, discounted pharmacy networks, mail service pharmacies, and more efficient (paperless) claims processing became major services offered by the PBMs.

PBM Services

Today, clients want the next level of cost efficiency—lowering the cost of total health care—which requires more complex and strategic clinical interventions with prescribers.[52] Online connectivity to the prescriber's office is a method of intervention that occurs before the patient is given a prescription. Disease management programs also impact total health care costs. Currently, PBMs are scrambling to position themselves in this arena and are viewed as consultants on pharmacy benefits (see Table 9.7).

PBM Ownership Issues

PBMs fall into one of four categories of ownership: drug-manufacturer-owned, independent, MCO-owned, and drugstore-chain-owned. A recent controversy

125

Table 9.7

Services Offered by Pharmacy Benefit Management Companies (PBMs)

- electronic/paper claims processing
- mail service pharmacy
- clinical management
- formulary
- rebates or discounts
- provider education
- management reporting
- pharmacy networks
- disease management
- benefit consulting
- sales and marketing training
- data integration
- member and provider service
- consulting services

that drew national attention relates to the manufacturer-owned PBMs and centers on whether vertical integration presents a conflict of interest. The FDA stated its plans to regulate the advertising and marketing of manufacturer-owned PBMs by mid-1998.[53] FDA's key concern: Do drug-switching practices occur for financial reasons only? In recent years, manufacturer-owned PBMs successfully contributed to the market share growth of their parent companies. Proposed regulation may slow aggressive switching activities.

The Future for PBMs

Health care payers will continue to purchase the basic PBM services. However, the consolidation and emergence of a more sophisticated PBM may result in few firms solely offering commodity services, such as claims processing and pharmacy network management. Clinically based PBMs must continue integrating medical information to focus on total care management. Critical success factors for a PBM include customer service, technology, benefit consulting, strong clinical programs, and the ability to work at the total care management level. PBMs that rely heavily on manufacturer rebates for their financial success may not survive.[54]

"Carve-Outs" vs. Integrated Pharmacy Programs

As PBMs evolved, there was a tendency to "carve-out" the prescription drug portion of the health care benefit for more effective management. By carving-out the benefit, employer groups and health plans pay the PBM a per capita amount to take advantage of discounted pharmacy networks, manufacturer rebate programs, clinical management programs, and more sophisticated reporting. However, if a PBM is financially responsible to manage drug expenditures, there is concern that the result may be medications that are inappropriate in regard to the patient's total care management. For example, if an expensive drug therapy enables a patient to move from inpatient to an ambulatory care setting, a financially at-risk PBM might resist the additional cost burden even though the prescription lowers total health care costs. This scenario illustrates the natural conflict that exists in the financial relationships of benefit carve-out programs, and argues for keeping pharmacy integrated with medical benefits. From a quality perspective, the integration of pharmacy and medical data creates powerful information to improve care for all members, whether the information originates in-house or through a carve-out.

◼ Conclusion

The future demands more aggressive patient management to focus on appropriate care across many benefit programs: medical, pharmacy, case management, demand management, behavioral health, disability, and workers' compensation. The need for accurate and timely information is critical to improve care for current patients.

Consolidation in the industry will continue for pharmaceutical manufacturers, PBMs, and health care organizations. Providers will become more sophisticated and closely linked to health plans. It appears that these providers also will be involved financially and that government regulators are likely to monitor these financial arrangements closely.[55] Pharmacy benefit programs underwent tremendous change during the last five years, and the pace will continue into the next century.

◼ Key Terms

"Carve-outs"
Average wholesale price (AWP)
Benefit design references
Clinical and administrative edits

Clinical management programs
Closed formulary
Customer service program
Disease management programs

Dispensing fee
Drug benefit management
Drug use evaluation (DUE)
Drug utilization reports

Drug utilization review (DUR)
Electronic claims processing
Generic drugs
Integrated pharmacy programs
Mail service pharmacy
NCQA/HEDIS
Open formulary
Patient profiling
"Pay for Performance" program
Pharmaceutical manufacturer discounts/rebates
Pharmacy and therapeutic (P&T) committee
Pharmacy benefit management company (PBM)
Pharmacy benefit plan reporting
Pharmacy care program
Pharmacy networks
Preferred formulary
Prescription drug formulary
Prior authorization
Processing performance standards
Provider profiling
Therapeutic interchange
Treatment guidelines
Universal Claim Form (UCF)

Chapter 10

MANAGED DENTAL CARE

■ Introduction

According to the National Institute of Dental Research (NIDR), America's dental health has never been better. The number of children without tooth decay increased from 26 percent in 1974 to 55 percent in 1991, and cavities between the teeth in children are a disappearing problem.[56] The combination of dental insurance, fluoridated water supplies, fluoride treatments, better oral hygiene, and more visits to the dentist enables people to retain their teeth longer. *Health Care Financing Review* reports that the cost of dental care, at $45.8 billion in 1995, represents only 5.2 percent of personal health care expenditures.[57] However, expenditures for dental services are increasing at a greater rate than expenditures for either hospitals or physicians.

Because people are keeping their teeth longer than previous generations did, more teeth are at risk for dental disease later in life. Increasingly, tooth decay and periodontal disease are becoming diseases of mature adulthood. NIDR reported that 63 percent of mature adults had decay on exposed roots and 34 percent had severe periodontal disease.[58] Dr. Chester Douglas of the Harvard School of Dental Medicine wrote, "The increase in need for adult operative dentistry is three times the decrease in need for children's operative dentistry," and, "The population growth combined with increased tooth retention, simply overwhelms the increase in the number of dentists." In the near future, the availability of dentists will be a challenge for managed care plans.

The National Association of Dental Plans (NADP) reports that 45 percent of the population is covered by dental benefits. NADP estimates that the number of persons with dental coverage increased from 117 million in 1995 to 124 million in 1996, from 45.7 percent of the total population to 46.7 percent. Growth of dental HMOs is forecast as 15 percent, to a total of 23.9 million members. And growth of dental PPOs is estimated at 20 percent, to a total of 17 million members. Of those with dental benefits, 74 percent are in the private market and 26 percent under Medicaid, military, and other government programs.[59] The American Dental Association's (ADA) 1996 Survey of Dental Practice reports that 63 percent of dentists' patients have private dental insurance and 5 percent receive benefits under government programs.[60] These data strongly suggest that people who are covered by dental insurance are encouraged to visit the dentist.

▇ Dental is Different

There are significant differences between dentistry and general medicine. The medical model cannot be used as a model for dental care. Knowing these differences is important to the design and administration of a dental model for managed care.

Dental Insurance

Dental insurance is not insurance in the classic sense. Most health insurance has a high-loss severity with low frequency: Most people are not hospitalized in any given year, but those who are hospitalized incur high costs. Dental disease is exactly the opposite: There is a high frequency (the overwhelming majority of the population has some dental disease) and low-loss severity (most dental disease is treated at a much lower cost than medical illness or injuries).

Dentists

Sixty-nine percent of dentists practice alone, another 20 percent practice with one other dentist, and only 12 percent are involved in a group practice (percentages are rounded). Eight percent of dentists are employees. Since 1983, solo practitioners decreased by 6 percent, those working with one other dentist increased by 12 percent, those working in a group practice increased by 22 percent, and dentists who are employees increased by 46 percent.[61]

In dentistry, the gatekeeper concept already exists. Eighty percent of dentists are in general practice, in contrast to their medical colleagues where only 34 percent are engaged in primary care. This may explain why dental patients rarely "self-refer" to a dental specialist. Patients usually develop a close relationship with their "family" dentist, visiting frequently for routine check-ups. Rarely are dental visits a matter of life and death.

Dentists are not nearly as active in managed care as physicians. Eighty-eight percent of physicians participate in managed care, compared with less than 50 percent of dentists. Only 19 percent of dentists participate in dental heath maintenance (managed care) organizations (DHMO), compared with more than 33 percent who participate in preferred provider organizations (PPOs).

Prevention, Diagnosis, and Treatment

In dentistry, prevention works and is cost effective. Fluoride treatments, fluoridated water supplies, and toothpaste are proven to be very cost effective. These items saved millions of dollars in treatment cost—far more than the cost of the preventive procedures themselves. Early treatment is cost effective because costs increase when treatment is delayed.

In medicine, there are countless different disease entities and variations. Dental treatment applies primarily to two diseases: tooth decay and periodontal (gum) disease. Whereas medical diagnosis can be difficult, costly, and time-consuming, in dentistry, diagnosis and treatment are far more standardized and less varied. An examination by a dentist usually consists of a visual examination and, when indicated, X-rays. The use of expensive technologies during routine examinations is rare.

Practice Locations

In comparison with physicians, dentists operate very independently. With the exception of severely handicapped patients and a few oral surgical procedures, very little of dentistry requires hospitalization. Physicians in managed care must affiliate with a hospital if they are to provide comprehensive care. Dentists provide almost all services covered by dental plans in their own offices or the office of a specialist.

Treatment Options

Often, dentistry offers alternative methods of treatment for the same condition: a good, better, and best method. All treatments may be professionally acceptable, and all have different costs. Dental plans usually limit their liability to the "least expensive (professionally acceptable) alternate treatment," or LEAT. For example, if a silver amalgam satisfactorily fills a tooth, the plan pays for the cost of a silver amalgam, not for a more expensive gold inlay or crown. When patients prefer a gold filling, they pay the difference in cost between silver and gold. This method of reimbursement is detailed in an alternate treatment clause in the plan document and summary plan description.

■ Managed Dental Care

The various types of managed care plans in the dental model include:

Dental MCO

A dental MCO is a capitated plan, whereby dentists are paid on a per capita basis at a fixed (usually monthly) rate for each individual or family. The dentist is paid irrespective of the number or types of services provided or the number of beneficiaries seen. The dentist is at financial risk for the enrollees' utilization.

Staff Model

A dental plan with one or more dental offices that uses salaried (staff) dentists, the staff model works successfully with capitation plans. It may be a closed panel operated by the entity providing services for its own beneficiaries or a contracted dental office(s) that provides services to one or more purchasers.

Network Model

A dental plan with multiple dental offices in various locations, this is the most common method of delivering dental benefits in a dental HMO or PPO. The offices may be limited to a specific geographic area or spread over many states. The administrator usually contracts with private dental offices, principally fee-for-service dental practices.

Preferred Provider Organizations (PPOs)

In a PPO, a network of dentists contracts to accept a specific level of payment for providing covered services. Dentists are paid on a fee-for-service basis either with discounted reasonable and customary fees or under a fee schedule (fixed-fee PPO). The dentist is not at risk (see key differences between dental HMOs and dental PPOs in Table 10.1).

Table 10.1

Key Considerations between Dental Plan Types

Factor	Dental HMOs	Dental PPOs
Critical mass	Enough lives must be enrolled in a dental office to reduce the risk to the dentist: the minimum is about 100. A dentist with only a few patients under capitation payment of $10 per month per member loses substantial money if a patient needs extensive work—unless guarantees exist to protect against loss or enough lives are enrolled.	"Critical mass" is not as important and the dentist is not at risk. The dentist is paid a fee for each service provided: the more services the greater the income. Depending on patient volume or the fee schedule, they may decline additional PPO patients or ask to participate only for patients of record.
Recruitment	Dentists are busier and some decline to join a dental HMO. In 1997 only 18 percent of dentists participated in dental HMOs. Group practices, new dentists and DPMCs are the principal entities willing to provide care for dental HMOs.	Dentists prefer payment on a fee-for-service basis. As a form of managed care, a dental PPO more closely mirrors the traditional way of practicing dentistry. The risk of anti-selections that exist in a dental HMO is absent.
Offices	It is difficult to have numerous offices participate in an area because it reduces the number of lives delivered to each office. To provide dentists with a "critical mass" of lives and have an office "on every corner" is rarely achievable.	Because critical mass is not as important and recruitment is easier, more dental offices are likely to participate given a reasonable fee schedule.
Development expense	Dental HMO networks are expensive to develop, especially multi-state networks. To recruit a quality network requires multiple office visits, thorough credentialing, personal relationships with each office, and periodical onsite reviews.	Dentists participating in dental PPO networks usually enroll by mail. It is rare to need an office visit to discuss how a dental PPO operates. This makes a dental PPO network considerably less expensive to develop.
Financially advantageous	If managed care doesn't work for the dentist, it won't work. It is essential to select dental offices that are well managed and to reimburse adequately for services provided.	Fee schedules are generally targeted at the 50th percentile. At that level, one half of all procedures reported are paid in full. Nothing overcomes a low fee schedule. Expecting to receive services for less than cost simply does not work. The dentist needs to cover costs—and earn a profit.
Copayments	A 50% (minimum) copayment for major services encourages patient cooperation—essential for a successful outcome. Without good oral hygiene, the most expensive bridge or the best treatment for periodontal disease soon fails and necessitate a repeat procedure at an additional cost. In such situations, the better dental HMO and fee-for-service plans offer an exclusion for payment and the patient must pay for the additional treatment.	Same as for dental HMO. Patients often fail to do their part when they lack a financial stake in the outcome.

continued

133

Table 10.1 (*Continued*)

Factor	Dental HMOs	Dental PPOs
Comprehensive utilization data	Comprehensive data on plan performance is not an option, it is essential to make intelligent observations, decisions, or plans and to identify problems. The best and most cost-effective way to identify dentists who practice less than appropriate dentistry is with comprehensive utilization reports that detail what they provide compared with their peers—then take corrective action.	Same as for DHMO
Incentives	In a well-designed dental HMO there are two ways for a dentist to make money: bring patients to a good level of oral health maintenance or do as little as possible. With patients on maintenance the dentist only has to do recalls and an occasional service. This is the ideal situation. But some dental offices discourage patient visits through long waits for an appointment, long time between appointments, and long waits at the dental office, and then provide only one or two services per visit. Geographically inaccessible offices are another barrier to deter patients. One office even went to the extreme of routinely giving painful injections to discourage patients from seeking treatment.	The incentive to treat or over-treat exists in all fee-for-service dental plans. Dentists may make up for "discounted fees" by upgrading (i.e., reporting a $40 dollar teeth cleaning as a $150 scaling and root planing) or by providing more expensive services than necessary to maintaining dental health (i.e., using a $500 crown when a $60 silver amalgam filling would adequately restore the tooth). That is why utilization review data are important.

Dental Practice Management Companies (DPMCs) or Dental Service Organizations (DSOs)

A DPMC or DSO may or may not be owned by dentists. DPMCs typically buy a dental practice(s) and retain the dentist(s) on a salaried and/or commission basis to provide care. The DPMC or DSO manages all business aspects of the practice, allowing the dentists to spend their full time treating patients. These management services are also available to dentists who maintain ownership of their practice, under an agreement with a DPMC or DSO.

◼ Minimum Data Requirements

Managed care requires a comprehensive information system to support compliance with the health plans, monitor performance and trends, and efficiently and accurately manage finances. Specific data requirements include:

Data Capture

Data collection should include a summary of services provided and their value. Data for all services from all types of dental plans should be captured. Data elements should include the ADA code, frequency, charge, and allowance. Data should be available by patient, dentist, and aggregated by account.

Reports

Comprehensive reports on services and value are especially valuable in dental MCOs, because it is important to determine whether value is received for the premiums paid.

Analysis and Audit

Details of treatment are important to determine whether practice patterns fall within the norms of dental practice. For example, do extractions and examinations exceed teeth cleaning? If so, something is probably wrong.

In addition to internal analysis, an independent audit of data is necessary. Dentists and plan administrators, perhaps unintentionally, may not be objective in their analysis of reports on quality, value, and overall performance. It is essential that independent audits be conducted on all dental plans.

■ Ten Realities to Consider When Establishing a Dental Managed Care Network

1. The dental plan must work for the dentist or it is destined to fail. Dental offices that are well managed and dedicated to quality care must be treated fairly regarding compensation, with a minimum of bureaucracy.

2. Managed dental care is a complex business. Individuals who view managed dental care as a "simple" product are destined to make many costly mistakes. This is especially true for those who do not understand the differences between the dental and medical models.

3. Dental HMOs must protect the dentist from serious financial loss. It is essential for the plan administrator who priced and sold the plan to protect the dentist from serious loss. The dentist, lacking the resources to retain actuaries and MBAs to evaluate the risk, depends on the administrator for financial protection.

4. Although dentists need protection from serious financial loss, they must share in the risk. Without risk, a dentist may over-treat or provide unnecessary treatment.

135

5. Dental networks are more difficult to establish than medical networks. Dentists today are busier than in the past and are more resistant to joining MCOs. Careful attention must be paid to plan design and compensation to ensure that there are enough dentists to provide care.

6. Dentists join networks to increase/maintain a patient base and increase/maintain their income. Lacking these incentives, it is difficult, if not impossible, to build a network.

7. When all efforts fail, administrators may need to establish a dental facility. Lacking the sufficient number of lives to make this financially feasible, the administrator must consider options, such as an interest-free loan to a dentist willing to locate in the area of need.

8. Group practices that provide both a full range of dental services and economies of scale, and can afford a full-time business manager, will become the backbone of managed care.

9. Excessive retentions spell "trouble." Retention is that portion of the premium the administrator uses for profit and administrative cost, with the remainder going to dentists for dental services. Dental HMO premiums are lower than indemnity plans, but the cost of administration is not necessarily less. Although the percentage of retention will be higher than in more costly indemnity plans, it should be kept as low as possible.

10. Plan design is the key to cost management and dentist satisfaction. It is essential to have a well-written plan that clearly spells out what is, and is not, covered. For example, if the plan does not contain a LEAT limitation, the dentist in the dental HMO and the plan in a dental PPO (DPPO) may suffer significant financial losses.

■ The Future for Managed Dental Care

A number of challenges face dental managed care. They include:

Availability of Dentists

Diminishing Numbers

Because of decreased numbers and increasingly busier dentists who (as the sellers of services) control the market, the supply of dentists willing to participate in managed care may be limited.

Shrinking Dental School Enrollment

While medicine is now asking questions about a possible oversupply of physicians, dentistry addressed the issue of oversupply in the 1970s. The number of dental schools grew from 42 with 3,200 first-year students in 1950 to 60 dental schools with 6,300 first-year students in 1978. But since then, the number of schools and students has decreased significantly. In 1998 there were 56 schools with 4,200 first-year students. Some authorities believe that the number of dental graduates is insufficient to meet the growing need and demand for dental care. By way of comparison, from 1965 to 1985 the number of physicians increased 85 percent while the number of dentists increased only 33 percent.

Views of Women Dentists

The views of women dentists about full- and part-time employment also has an impact on the supply of dentists. In 1976, women constituted 14 percent of first-year enrollees in dental schools. By 1996 that number increased to 38 percent, and some predictions are for women to constitute 50 percent of dental students by the year 2000. In a survey conducted by the American Dental Association, however, only 29 percent of women said full-time work was very important, compared with 45 percent of men. Similarly, 32 percent of women said working part time was very important, compared with 11 percent of men.[62]

The combination of a decrease in the number of dental graduates, more women pursuing dentistry as a part-time profession, and an increasing demand for dental care makes it more difficult to recruit dentists to participate in managed dental care plans. On the other hand, these circumstances may increase the availability of dentists who wish to practice part time for DPMCs or DSOs. A study by the American Dental Association reported that women and recent graduates are more likely to participate in managed care plans than their older male colleagues. Furthermore, dentists may need to participate in a health plan because many of their patients have central coverage that requires such participation.

Selective Contracting

The principal driver of cost in a dental plan is the type and frequency of service. Dental care's largest costs are incurred for crowns and permanent bridges. On a national basis, these items constitute 27 percent of charges. Dentists who are moderate in their use of these services will become the winners in this mode of managed care. In the future, PPOs that contract with cost-effective providers are likely to experience the most growth.

Dental Practice Management Companies (DPMCs)

The growth of DPMCs in the last several years is significant and is expected to continue. Many DPMCs are now publicly traded, and many have been created principally to service the managed care industry. Consolidation in the industry is likely to continue.

Electronic Data Interchange

Electronic submission of claims and X-rays reduces administrative cost and simplifies claims submission for dentists and administrators, makes claims payments and review more cost effective, and enables the dentist to retain the original X-rays. Increasingly, government oversight of health care will encompass dental care and result in mandated electronic submission of claims and X-rays.

Quality of Care Measurement

The National Committee for Quality Assurance (NCQA) has standards for dental care provided through affiliation with a medical MCO. The National Association of Dental Plans is currently addressing the issue of quality standards for dental HMOs.

■ Conclusion

Over the past few years, the total of lives covered has remained relatively steady, but more benefits have been provided through dental HMO plans. Two-thirds of the companies that rely on traditional employee dental benefit plans predict that they will switch to dental managed care plans in the near future.[63]

■ Key Terms

Alternate treatment
Copayment
Critical mass
Dental health
  maintenance
  organization (DHMO)
Dental practice
  management company
  (DPMC)

Dental preferred
  provider organization
  (DPPO)
Dental service
  organization (DSO)
Electronic submission
Gatekeeper
Least expensive
  alternate treatment
  (LEAT)

National Association of
  Dental Plans (NADP)
Network model
Periodontal disease
Quality of care
  measurement
Staff model
Utilization

Chapter 11

BEHAVIORAL HEALTH PROGRAMS

■ Introduction

Widespread and rapid changes occurred in the practice of medicine during the 1990s. In the past, medical changes were synonymous with innovations in diagnostic and therapeutic technologies. The recent changes, however, impact the architectural structure of health care delivery systems. Although technological advances continue to affect changes in practice patterns, nothing has influenced the practice of medicine (especially psychiatry) more than the explosion in managed care.

Managed care in a variety of forms is here to stay, despite opposition from providers. Some, like Mark Alan Thompson, M.D., suggest that physicians have contributed to the change. In a letter to the *New England Journal of Medicine* he writes, "But we forfeited the moral high ground long ago when we let our own desire for private enrichments displace our commitment to service through the alleviation of suffering, especially care of the poor. We sold out. Instead of choosing patient care as our preeminent concern, we cultivated a cottage industry of moneymaking that sooner or later would be ripe for a takeover."[64]

Dr. Thompson's viewpoint that managed care reflects a "takeover" is one of a number of obstacles that an MCO must overcome to provide behavioral health services. Opposition from providers toward managed care arises from the fact that managed care's financial incentives alter typical practice patterns. Managed care mechanisms—such as utilization management protocols that aim at rapidly administered and shorter lengths of treatments, accountability for the coordination of care, and consultation for treatment options—result in changes in traditional practice.

▨ Obstacles to Managed Care

To meet enrollees' needs for behavioral health care, an MCO must create an integrated network of services. In behavioral health, that becomes complicated because of the obstacles encountered as a result of the current approach to delivering these services. Some obstacles are:

Cottage Industry Delivery Approach

Dr. Thompson is accurate in applying the term "cottage industry"—a prevalence of small, individualized units of providers and services—to traditional health care. The term, however, no longer describes how medical/surgical care is provided in most of this country. It *is* still descriptive of behavioral health care, where shared clinical practices exist only in limited settings. For example, in training institutes and clinics, care is rendered by multidisciplinary teams, with psychiatrists serving as consultants or team leaders. Such analytic institutes and other training forums afford situations for group supervision or group dialogue on cases. Unfortunately, such group "think tanks" cease once providers enter into full-time private practices.

Prevalence of Individual Provider Model

MCOs require the provision of health care services to a large population with multiple treatment needs. The individual provider model is outmoded for the delivery of medical/surgical and behavioral health care under managed care. Medical and surgical practices more readily lend themselves to the group and multidisciplinary systems that oversee volume practices, multiplicity of disorders, and access and emergency coverage. These same requirements exist for behavioral health services, but implementation problems are compounded for behavioral health by the prevalence of the solo practitioner model and by providers who work literally "behind closed doors."

Unknown Practice Quality

Patients confer with behavioral health care providers for all kinds of disorders. Unfortunately, providers customarily offer or recommend those treatments with which they are most familiar, and not necessarily the treatment modality that has the greatest degree of specificity for the illness in question. To address this dilemma, numerous organizations, including the American Psychiatric Association, American Association of Addiction Medicine, and American Behavioral Healthcare Association, develop and promote the use of practice guidelines.

Another crucial step is the improvement of clinicians' training so that they develop expertise in a number of treatment modalities.

A lack of routine scrutiny of one's treatment cases leads to an insular treatment environment. One contributing factor involves patient confidentiality. As a consequence, two major problems arise:

■ The monitoring of the progress and outcome of behavioral health treatment is greatly compromised.

■ A stigmatization and mystification of the behavioral health field is perpetuated, to the detriment of all concerned.

Resistance to Innovation

The behavioral health care field is not known for many technical innovations in treatment. For example, only recently did training institutes fully support research and development in short-term treatment modalities. Similarly, professionals in the field disagree about the use of even minor technical advances such as videotaping psychotherapy sessions for training, supervision, and patient teaching purposes. At the heart of the issue is a lack of support for research and training for significant treatment alternatives.

Confidentiality Barriers

Behavioral health care providers have often used the issue of patient confidentiality to obfuscate the need to monitor treatment. The persistent argument that scrutiny of behavioral health treatments infringes upon patient confidentiality contributes to the continued stigma and mystique that are often associated with behavioral health services. Behavioral health professionals can put this argument to rest by adopting policies that uphold confidentiality without impeding efforts to monitor and measure treatment selection, progress, and outcomes.

■ Creating an Integrated System

In the United States, medical and behavioral health care practices have concentrated on care provided by one entity in the continuum, such as a hospital or an ambulatory setting. For example, a psychiatric hospital views its role as performing a programmatic regimen, after which the patient is discharged. It may receive minimal input regarding:

■ the patient's past medical and psychiatric treatment history;

■ any consideration of financial expenditures; or

■ an exploration of alternative levels of step-down care.

In contrast, the care management activities in an MCO regard as significant the transition from one level of care to another, recognizing the powerful impact of each component on the one that follows. MCOs focus attention on the longer-term condition of the patient, not just the immediate resolution of a problem.

The current challenge for the MCO is to create an integrated system of behavioral health services that can demonstrate effectiveness both in controlling costs and improving health. MCOs seek to establish a vertically integrated health care system as a means to offer the most comprehensive and, therefore, cost-efficient care. When fully operational, the system delivers the right care, at the right time, in the right setting. A precondition for this success is the creation of various health care systems that provide consumers with a choice, as well as specialized differences in the services.

Service Components

To meet the MCO challenge, behavioral health providers must develop an integrated delivery system with the ability to track and coordinate services throughout the unitary components of a full "continuum of care." In behavioral health, a full continuum refers to the following structural or functional components of a vertically integrated network:

- inpatient facility
- partial or day hospital
- residential treatment facility
- intensive outpatient care
- structured outpatient chemical dependency programs
- emergency evaluations and treatment
- urgent and routine care
- ancillary services
- home care
- coordination of care with the primary care physician

Collaboration and Integration

An integrated delivery system means that formal collaboration must exist among providers through mergers, affiliations, and expansion of services. For example, to integrate or expand services, providers can:

■ convert independent hospital facilities into full-service entities that offer many levels of care; or

■ create multidisciplinary group practices that combine the solo practices of several behavioral health professionals under a single management.

New Skills

The changes brought on by managed care may lead behavioral health care providers to think that the rules changed and that, under the new rules, they lack the skills to succeed. Working in a managed care environment does require a new skill set. It is critical for behavioral health care providers to actively participate in the design and management of the services offered within a vertically integrated system. To function effectively, they first must demonstrate expertise in:

■ care management functions, particularly in the most debilitated patient populations;

■ preventive medicine;

■ disease management programs;

■ practice guidelines development;

■ outcomes measurement research;

■ quality improvement methods;

■ coordination/integration of behavioral health care with primary medical care; and

■ medical finances.

Armed with expertise in these disciplines, behavioral health care professionals can contribute to the success of an integrated delivery system. Their expertise and active involvement is critical to the performance of the accountability functions within MCOs.

■ Accountability and Quality

Once removed from the training setting, providers must attend meetings and seminars to earn the continuing educational credits required to maintain their licenses. It is difficult for an MCO to determine whether (or how much) continuing education or research influence a practitioner's treatment process when the care is rendered by a solo practitioner who lacks any external motivation or oversight.

The creation of an integrated system with full accountability will take time, but economic forces demand new approaches. Therefore, business as usual will not suffice. MCOs are in an optimal position to collaborate with behavioral health professionals to develop new approaches. In the meantime, MCOs must use available tools that can help to measure quality and utilization of the individual services. The MCOs' goal is to establish best practices as standard business throughout their behavioral health care networks. Frequently used tools include:

Provider Profiles

Provider profiles are one element of a quality improvement process for behavioral health. They serve as an instrument for provider feedback. Profiling reports compare a provider or a facility with a peer group along a number of parameters. In behavioral health, profiles have not been widely used because of a lack of access to information and problems with the uniformity of data. These difficulties limit an MCO's profiling elements to:

- utilization statistics;
- adherence to access and availability standards;
- patient satisfaction;
- medical record integrity;
- coordination of care accountability; and
- adherence to practice guidelines (when they exist).

Practice Guidelines

Practice guidelines facilitate clinical decision making in medical and surgical practices. Behavioral health care guidelines, although still new in the field, are being heavily promulgated. Providers must become familiar with the practice guidelines and various disease treatment algorithms of each MCO and provide feedback to health plans regarding those guidelines that do and do not work. The National Committee for Quality Assurance (NCQA) scores MCOs on how well they promote provider participation in the development of practice guidelines. That should encourage MCOs and providers to collaborate to develop effective guidelines. Once a guideline is accepted as a best practice, it can be fairly used as a measure of a clinician's performance.

Outcome Studies

Outcome measures are likely to be the richest and most complicated area of study for both psychiatric and substance abuse disorders. As a linchpin in

144

health care delivery, outcome measures maintain a focus on whether or not (and how much) improvement is made in the health care of the population served. Outcomes research is a rapidly expanding area of medical literature, and will have a profound effect on how psychotherapy is delivered in the future.

Accreditation

Behavioral health care organizations that are surveyed and accredited by the NCQA are measured for compliance with the same accreditation standards that are applied to medical services, including:

- quality improvement;
- utilization management;
- access, availability, and triage;
- members' rights and responsibilities;
- credentialing and re-credentialing;
- treatment records; and
- preventive behavioral health.

■ Conclusion

A paradigm shift is occurring in the provision of health care aimed at disease prevention and management programs. As the industry improves its capacity to contain the acute and subacute phases of disorders, resources are increasingly directed toward prevention. Identifying at-risk populations and creating out-reach programs to address early detection and intervention are significant issues for medical and behavioral health care.

To move forward, behavioral health professionals must address an existing insidious attitude, one that is skeptical of change and innovation. If this attitude prevails, the credibility of the behavioral health therapies will be damaged and a pervasive public mistrust of the field will grow. To ensure behavioral health's future role in determining how, when, and which services are provided, professionals must:

- acknowledge the obstacles that exist in the current system;
- commit resources for outcomes research to refine which disorders respond to which treatment protocols;
- devote energy to develop and test new treatment options;

- offer expert training in traditional and innovative treatment techniques such as family therapies and short-term therapies;
- create an integrated approach to the delivery of services through group practices, affiliations, and other formal arrangements; and
- gain the skills necessary to provide leadership in a managed care system.

■ Key Terms

Accreditation
Cottage industry
Integrated delivery
   system

Outcome studies
Practice guidelines
Provider profiles
System delivery

Treatment options
Vertically integrated
   network

Chapter 12

VISION CARE PROGRAMS

■ Introduction

Vision and eye health conditions are the second most prevalent chronic problem in the United States, and 60 percent of Americans are currently in need of vision correction. In 1995, the optical retail market amounted to an estimated $13.6 billion. Despite these already staggering numbers, the demand for vision care services is expected to grow rapidly during the first decade of the new century. With the "aging of America" phenomenon, many individuals with good eyesight throughout their childhoods and early adult years will require vision correction during the mid- and later-life stages. In addition to medical eye care conditions common among the elderly, presbyopia (in which the eye loses its ability to focus sharply on close objects, creating the need for bifocals) affects many individuals in their mid-40s and beyond. As baby boomers mature, the number of Americans estimated to need corrective eyewear is projected to grow at a rate of over one million people annually through 2011.

Significant growth in the vision care and corrective eyewear market can also be attributed to advances in corrective eyewear products. New and varied product offerings make eyewear more convenient, more comfortable, more attractive, and more adaptable to people's varied lifestyles. Consumers' perception of eyewear changes: An item that was purely functional becomes something that is fashionable, makes a personality statement, and is generally desirable.

■ Vision Care's Role in Managed Health Care

Prior to the emergence of managed health care, individuals traditionally purchased vision care services out-of-pocket with little or no insurance coverage.

However, the evolving emphasis on wellness and preventive care dramatically impacts the financing of vision care services.

Unique Service

Vision care is unique among health care services in several respects.

- It is the only component of health care that has a fashion element.

- It is the only component of health care that delivers a tangible product, other than medical supplies, hearing aids, etc. (all of which serve a medical function, but none of which are sought after, as is eyewear).

- It is one of few health care services that members do not have to be sick to use.

- Routine vision care is most often a one- or two-time painless encounter without ongoing treatment.

- Although many eye care providers practice in traditional, private-practice settings, vision care is also available in a retail setting (shopping malls, department stores, and discount consumers' clubs). Retail-based providers can be found in both small, local/regional groups with one or more practitioners and large, national chain stores. Consumer research indicates a higher level of patient satisfaction among services provided by private practitioners' offices over retail outlets. In contrast, many patients prefer the more convenient hours and locations of retail centers and perceive them as less intimidating than the traditional medical setting. The choice is highly personal, and both delivery modes are in demand.

Disease Detection

Routine eye exams aid in the early detection of a number of medical conditions, such as cancer, hypertension, diabetes, and glaucoma, even if a person is not experiencing any other related symptoms.

Growing Popularity

For all of these reasons, vision care is a "feel good" benefit whose positive emotional context ensures its popularity among recipients of group benefits. Consider these findings from a study of more than 1,000 working adults. Seventy-three percent of respondents felt that employers should offer vision benefits, and 61 percent of those polled felt so strongly that they would trade a vacation day for coverage of an eye exam and glasses.[65]

Vision benefits are growing in popularity among MCOs as they seek ways to boost market share by offering popular benefits not offered by their competitors. Vision coverage is added to a benefits package at a relatively small cost compared with more complex and expensive benefits (such as mental health and prescription drugs), adding to its popularity with plan decision-makers.

■ Levels of Vision Care

We must distinguish between the various care levels encompassed by vision and eye care benefits.

Routine Vision Care

The most basic level of care is wellness or routine vision care, which includes a routine eye examination to determine general eye health and the need for visual correction. Although coverage of this service is less common than medical and surgical eye care services, it is gaining popularity. A recent study of 1,500 employer and trust fund administrators, each with 5,000+ covered lives, found that of all benefit options considered for addition to benefits packages, vision care is expected to have the greatest growth. When covered, routine vision benefits generally include a comprehensive eye examination once every 12 or 24 months, and sometimes include coverage of eyewear, ranging from simple discounts to modest or even generous allowances on eyewear purchases. Routine vision services are generally accessed by patients "on demand" (without referral), and plan eligibility is the sole criterion for coverage.

Medical Eye Care

The second level of care is nonsurgical medical eye care, which encompasses treatment of eye conditions such as conjunctivitis and glaucoma and the removal of foreign bodies. Since these services are directly medical in nature, benefit coverage is standard under almost all managed care plans.

Medical eye care services are either diagnostic (to confirm the presence of and identify an eye care condition) or therapeutic (treatment of the eye condition). Each state determines the breadth of services rendered by each type of eye care provider (optician, optometrist, ophthalmologist). In recent years, the scope of treatment privileges granted to optometrists has increased dramatically. Many managed care plans now utilize both optometrists and ophthalmologists for the delivery of services traditionally provided by ophthalmologists. Some managed health care plans—particularly those using a primary care physician gatekeeper model—require a referral or plan authorization for nonsurgical medical eye care. Other plans allow basic medical eye care services to be accessed "on demand" and reserve authorization requirements only for surgical services.

Surgical Eye Care

The most advanced level of eye care encompasses surgical procedures, most of which must be performed by an ophthalmologist. However, there is a growing trend of "co-management" by optometrists and ophthalmologists, whereby the optometrist renders pre- and post-surgical services and the ophthalmologist performs the actual surgical procedure. Surgical eye care services in the managed health care environment almost always require prior authorization by the plan and are often closely case-managed by the plan's utilization management staff.

■ Vision Benefit Managers

As with many ancillary benefits, MCOs increasingly delegate the management and administration of their vision and eye care programs to specialty organizations known as vision benefits managers (VBMs). This delegation or "carve-out" enhances the MCO in two ways.

- First, it relieves the MCO of the administrative burden of operating the program, allowing the plan to devote its usually limited resources to the management of higher-cost health care services.

- Second, most VBMs administer vision programs exclusively, are experts in vision care, and cover a high volume of lives. Therefore, the VBM has better bargaining power with providers and suppliers. The result is a lower cost structure for the plan, compared with the direct contracting alternative.

Most VBMs perform a full range of program management functions, including network development/provider relations, services authorization, utilization management, claims adjudication, member services, and utilization reporting/encounter data provision. VBMs also perform continuous quality improvement, which encompasses provider credentialing/re-credentialing, grievance research/resolution, member and provider satisfaction surveys, provider audits, and quality assurance studies.

Delegation of program management by a health plan to a VBM is structured in two ways:

■ Capitated carve-out

Under this most common method, the health plan pays a capitated rate to the VBM based on the benefit design and population demographics, in exchange for the assumption of claims risk by the VBM.

■ Management services

As an alternative, a health plan elects to retain financial responsibility for vision claims and pays the VBM an administrative fee for its program management services.

■ Provider Considerations

Practitioner Types

As previously mentioned, there are three types of eye care practitioners: opticians, optometrists, and ophthalmologists. Each differs in training and in the services they legally may provide.

Opticians: make and dispense eyewear. Some states permit opticians to conduct their business without licensure. Some also permit opticians to render a limited number of professional services, but, as a general rule, opticians are providers of eyewear, not services.

Optometrists: are licensed practitioners with four years of graduate training specific to eye care. Optometrists perform eye examinations, and most dispense eyewear. The exact breadth of services rendered by optometrists varies by state; however, nearly all states permit optometrists to perform some level of diagnostic and therapeutic medical eye care services.

Ophthalmologists: are licensed physicians who specialize in eye care and related surgical procedures. While some dispense eyewear, many restrict their practices to medical eye care services.

All three provider types are utilized by MCOs. Some plans limit their provider panel to one or two types, for a variety of quality, cost, or other considerations. Other MCOs include all three in their panel to achieve broad member appeal.

Eyewear Fabrication

Many eye care providers stock prescription eyeglass lenses in their offices. Some are able to "edge" lenses to fit the eyeglass frame selected by a patient, prefer to use their own equipment, and may provide a faster turnaround time for patients. Other providers send all eyewear orders to an outside ophthalmic laboratory for fabrication and frame insertion.

Many MCOs and VBMs require use of a designated ophthalmic laboratory. Such arrangements allow the program administrator to maintain a uniform quality control standard and to exercise volume-based purchasing power. An outside laboratory benefits the provider by removing the responsibilities for any breakage that occurs during the edging/insertion process and for the acquisition cost of the lenses (most MCOs and VBMs that use a designated laboratory pay the lab directly for the cost of lenses).

■ Conclusion

The unique characteristics of vision and eye care services set them apart from other health care endeavors and create an attractive component of a managed health care benefits package. As MCOs continually seek to derive the most benefit from their premium dollars, they are streamlining the delivery of vision and eye care services through the integration of routine, medical, and surgical eye care services. The prevalence of eye conditions and consumer demand for benefits will make vision and eye care services an even more important coverage issue during the years ahead and will ensure the continued evolution of this benefit component.

■ Key Terms

Capitated carve-out	Medical eye care	Surgical eye care
Disease detection	Ophthalmologist	Unique service
Eyewear fabrication	Optician	Vision benefit managers
Fashion component	Optometrist	(VBMs)
Management services	Routine vision care	Vision care

Section IV

IMPROVING MCO OPERATIONS

Managers of managed care organizations must contend with a number of external forces (such as legislation and conflicting demands from multiple stakeholders) that influence their business practices. However, coping with outside challenges is only part of their job. Managers must also commit to continuously improve their businesses, and must constantly make critical adjustments to strengthen their organizations' marketplace position.

Chapter 13 defines the improvements that are key to a mutually productive relationship between MCOs and physicians. Chapter 14 describes the improvements required to effectively control costs through better patient care—improvements that include going beyond basic accreditation requirements to state-of-the-art programs such as disease management. Chapter 15 identifies the steps necessary to reengineer a managed care delivery system based on the needs of patients/members.

Chapter 13

MANAGED CARE AND THE PHYSICIAN TODAY

■ Introduction

Managed care evolved into the powerful force it is today largely because of decades of physicians' indifference to inflationary health care cost increases. Despite physician opposition, managed care has stemmed what many thought to be inexorable inflationary cost increases. During this same period, physicians contributed to a growing consumer backlash, lodging complaints about managed care's intrusion into aspects of clinical care that, traditionally, were entirely within the physician's domain.

Unfortunately, relations between MCOs and physicians became adversarial as MCOs engaged in vigorous price competition in response to purchasers' demands.[66] Perhaps much of the tension (or even overt hostility) that too often characterizes their relationship was inevitable as MCOs became more successful. However, to continue their success in the future, some MCOs will need to take steps to minimize the large cultural and economic gulf that exists between them and physicians. One such step is for MCOs to recognize that it is the physician—not the organization—that provides or orders most health care services and enjoys the primary allegiance of patients.

It is difficult to generalize about physicians, particularly in their responses to the profound changes in health care delivery represented by managed care. Some physicians now say they would tolerate a single government payer over

MCO intrusion. Conversely, other physicians are in the forefront of managed care developments and view market-based purchasing as an opportunity to demonstrate and be rewarded for the value of the services they provide.

Physicians participate in managed care in different ways. Originally, staff and group model health maintenance organizations (HMOs) relied on employed physicians with relations exclusive to one health plan. Since the late 1980s, managed care expansion (including both HMOs and PPOs [preferred provider organizations]) has moved away from this model. MCOs now rely on open-panel networks in which private practice physicians contract with many plans and lack strong allegiance to any particular one. The opening of physician panels and expansion of networks shifts the MCO and physician relationship into one of two approaches:

- a two-tier system in which the physician directly contracts with the MCO; or
- a three-tier system in which an individual practitioner, a medical group, or independent practice association (IPA) holds the MCO subcontract, thus creating three layers: individual physician, provider group, and health plan.

Most providers currently use a two-tier system, and the following discussion focuses on this arrangement.

■ Different Orientations

Despite its growth, managed care is not widely favored by the medical community. Actions to limit the control exercised by the MCO over provider decisions and patient choice are producing a deluge of legislation, by both federal and state governments. Underlying the complaints and opposition are fundamental differences in values and styles between MCOs and physicians. The MCO that works with its physicians to minimize these differences is likely to gain their commitment and cooperation. To begin, an MCO must understand these differences and recognize that physicians are not united in their views toward managed care.

Contrasts in Values

Some of the conflict between MCOs and physicians results from their strikingly different cultural and ethical orientations. Physicians are imbued with a culture of professionalism, as symbolized by these key tenets:

- Only similarly trained peers are capable of judging knowledge and competence.

Table 13.1

Different Core Attitudes and Behavior Patterns of Physicians and Managed Care Organizations (MCOs)

Physicians	MCOs
Provide medical care to individuals	Provide health care to populations
Focus on diagnosis and treatment of illness	Focus on prevention as well as diagnosis and treatment
Cost doesn't count or is secondary	Cost counts a lot
Quality is defined as practicing according to professional standards, and decisions about quality are applied to an individual patient	Quality is achieving improved outcomes for a population, and decisions about quality are based on and applied to a large group of patients
Accountability resides with an individual, autonomous physician	Accountability resides with an organization, in which physicians are part of the team

■ Knowledge and competence rest on a body of rational, scientific information that is kept current.

■ Physicians have an affirmative, ethical obligation to act in the best interests of their clients/patients who depend upon the professionals' submersion of their own self-interest.

In contrast, MCOs are products of marketplace competition and are oriented to customer and shareholder satisfaction. In well-functioning markets, quality and consumer well-being are protected through the ability of consumers to pick and choose among competitors (i.e., to vote with their feet). Consumers capable of discerning quality and price differences reward those sellers that provide the best value with their continued business. In most markets today, consumers lack the opportunity to select their preferred health delivery system, because employers select on behalf of their employees. This results in two customers: the purchaser who chooses the MCO, and the individual consumer of the MCO's services. At times, the interests and perceptions of purchasers and consumers may diverge, creating a conflict in mission for the MCO. Nevertheless, purchasers and consumers share some common interests (e.g., the cost of care, and the improvement of the employee/consumer's health).

Given the very different core attitudes and behavior patterns (Table 13.1), it is not surprising to find that relations between physicians and MCOs are often strained.

Even in a marketplace dominated by managed care, patients expect physicians and other medical professionals to demonstrate these core values and behaviors. They expect their health care professionals to assume personal responsibil-

157

ity for their well-being and to practice with high standards of integrity and competence. It is this expectation and their professional precepts that lead physicians to resist supervision and performance oversight. Professionals who are accustomed to the "captain of the ship" role may not adapt well to working in multidisciplinary teams. Finally, the anti-bureaucratic attitude predicated on benefits to individual patients often produces routine resistance toward any reasonable rule designed by an MCO to benefit the overall population it serves.

Age Variances

Physicians remain split in their response to the profound changes in health care delivery represented by managed care. While some physicians resist MCO intrusion in their practice, others actively participate in shaping managed care developments. To some extent, this disparity reflects age differences. The well-established physician—who trained decades ago and built a reputation and a sense of self-worth based on how well he or she performed as an independent professional with duties to individual patients—is less willing to accommodate to managed care. In contrast, the younger, recently trained physician better accepts managed care's orientation to population health, cost control, increasing reliance on non-physician health professionals, and active oversight of individual performance.

■ Market-Driven Arrangements

Practical developments in market competition also interfere with collaboration between physicians and MCOs. A competitive managed care marketplace is one with well-differentiated entities with features defined as clearly distinguishable: approaches to delivering care and unique networks of physicians, hospitals, and other providers. These features are difficult to realize or sustain under these market characteristics:

- Commercial purchasers, in response to their employees' desire for more providers, select insurance products with low price and broad physician choice.
- MCOs initiate contracts with private physicians in fairly loose, non-exclusive relationships. In many markets, formerly closed-panel MCOs now contract with private practice physicians and IPAs. PPOs expand their networks to include virtually all primary care physicians available in their market.
- To retain their patients, physicians feel pressured to join most plans in their market.
- Patients are not free to select the MCOs preferred by their physician, but are limited to those preferred by their employer.

Potentially, these conditions can unite physicians and MCOs to develop a strategy that meets the demands of both the marketplace and their patients. However, any strategy must negate the impact from the current approach which:

- decreases the MCO's ability to selectively contract with physician partners and, thus, limits its ability to distinguish itself in the marketplace through unique medical management approaches and programs; and

- compromises the physicians' ability to selectively contract with an MCO based on considerations such as its approach to medical management or its compensation package.

So far, these practical market realities have produced very large, somewhat unwieldy networks that respond to the consumer desire for provider choice, but interfere with collaboration between MCOs and physicians to improve the quality of the product.

■ Problems Impeding Collaboration

In addition to the market forces and values, there are problems in the implementation of managed care that impede collaboration between MCOs and physicians. These include:

Standardization of Operations

In exchange for participation in many networks, physicians want each MCO to manage health care in the same way, thus minimizing their administrative burden. However, standardization may impede cooperation and innovation. For example, physicians prefer consistent credentialing criteria and a single credentialing form, uniform payment policies, a common referral process, and identical processes and criteria for pre-authorization and utilization review. These preferences conflict with an MCO's need to differentiate itself and to introduce innovative programs and approaches to care in precisely those areas in which the physician seeks consistency. When mutual interests are served, MCOs can support standardization. However, MCOs should strive to be innovative when it serves a specific programmatic purpose and permits the health plan to differentiate itself in the market. Examples of program innovation include coverage of alternative medicine, easier access to specialists, and disease management programs (e.g., for asthma and diabetes). Unfortunately, even innovative programs may meet resistance because of physicians' preferences for their routine.

159

"Free-Riders"

Another impediment to MCO innovation is the so-called free-rider problem. An MCO that provides a relatively small percentage of a physician's practice is reluctant to invest resources to improve a physician's capacity to provide high quality, cost-effective care—especially when such an investment benefits its competitors' subscribers as much as its own. Even when activities are justified by their intrinsic contribution to improve patient care and indirectly improve the public's perception of managed care, the free-rider concern restrains MCO-initiated innovation.

Physician Buy-In

The practical reality is that physicians may resist even a well-intentioned, well-designed quality improvement program imposed by an MCO that provides only a low percentage of a physician's patients (a common situation). Without the incentive provided by a higher volume of patients or subscribers, it is difficult to gain the cooperation necessary to innovate. Therefore, MCOs should think hard about whether to follow the market trend toward broad provider networks that satisfy the purchasers' requests for greater provider choice.

PCPs vs. Specialists

Most MCOs orient their medical management programs to emphasize primary care, to the detriment of specialists. Typically, MCOs follow Medicare's lead and calibrate payments to increase the relative incomes of primary care physicians (PCPs) compared with those of specialists. Further, most MCOs and some PPOs use primary care case managers as gatekeepers to control patient access to other providers referred by the PCPs. The combined impact of physician income redistribution and the increased role of the PCP exacerbates underlying tensions between PCPs and specialists. In response to a basic complaint by patients against managed care, MCOs are retreating from the PCP-oriented delivery systems to provide easier access to specialists.

Academic Health Centers

Academic health centers (AHCs) are another party aggrieved by typical managed care policies and procedures. In the past, AHCs subsidized their extensive research and education activities, as well as their provision of under-compensated or charity care, by charging higher fees to commercial insurers and government payers. It is unreasonable to expect that, in a competitive environment, MCOs would voluntarily continue to subsidize education, research, and care to the uninsured—expenditures for what are essentially public goods. Instead, MCOs negotiate very aggressive payment rates for the hospital and specialized care provided by AHCs. The MCO utilizes market forces to pay academic physicians the same or similar rates as are paid to community physicians, despite additional teaching and research responsibilities. A practical consequence of this approach is AHC physicians' resentment of MCOs' "bottom-line" orientation.

Coverage Exclusions

The professional orientation of physicians often leads to contention over what MCO managers are likely to view as straightforward business decisions. For example, physicians often do not understand or accept as legitimate the difference between insurance and medical care, that is, that medical care that is desirable for the patient's well-being may not be covered under an insurance contract. Many coverage exclusions (e.g., for routine physical exams) make little sense to physicians concerned primarily with patients' health. In the past, physicians were never at risk for cost overruns and, therefore, never weighed the cost benefits of varying treatments. Accordingly, they consider many seemingly straightforward MCO requirements (e.g., formularies) as poorly thought out and intrusive.

■ Improving Relations with Physicians in a Two-Tier System

In the short run, plans have achieved success by squeezing reimbursement or capitation rates paid to physicians and by aggressive reviews for requested care. In the long run, the plans that work in a partnership with physicians are better positioned for success. Steps can be taken by the MCO to build stronger relations with its physicians. When applied consistently and firmly over a period of time, the following actions help overcome the problems stated above. These actions can lead to better relations with contracting physicians and a better managed care product for enrollees.[67]

Educate Physicians

MCOs need to help physicians to understand the difference between insurance and medical care. In many areas, physicians simply do not understand the rationale for managed care policies and the specific rules under which MCOs operate. For example, physicians often do not understand that a benefits contract may contain specific exclusions that the MCO is bound to enforce. Similarly, many physicians fail to understand that established rules exist to govern fee-for-service coding and payments. Physicians are intelligent, they understand data, and they respect their peers. MCO leadership can use these attributes to achieve behavioral changes that are consistent with its goals.

Although mailings, newsletters, and meetings can play vital communications roles, MCOs often fail to realize that physicians are overwhelmed with generic information from many sources. One-on-one education, by phone or letter, is a better strategy when a specific issue arises that captures the attention of a physician or office manager. Physicians and their staff appreciate a substantive explanation of the reasons why a service is not paid or a claim rejected, rather than a bureaucratic non-explanation. In addition, physicians do respond to data about their performance, especially when they can see comparisons with their peers.

Treat Physicians Fairly and Consistently

Treating physicians fairly and consistently, in accordance with contractual obligations, is a suggestion often made in the context of payment. For example, MCOs should pay clean claims in a timely fashion, and certainly within any time limits specified by contract or state law. It is important to consistently apply policies to re-price claims or adjust capitation rates for the demographic characteristics of the patients served.

This suggestion does not imply that physicians cannot be selected for targeted oversight (see below). Rather, such activity should be based on defensible, objective criteria that are impartially applied. It also does not imply that special deals cannot be cut with particular providers. After all, selective contracting is the essence of managed care.[68] The suggestion does mean that adherence to contracts is important.

Recognize the Risk Selection Problems Inherent in Capitation

Adjustments of payments to physicians and other providers should reflect the burden of illness presented by their capitated patients. Until validated, case-mix adjustment methodology is available, plans should strive to avoid some of the more egregious errors (for example, retrospectively assigning a hospitalized patient to a capitated provider, or failing to make capitation payments on behalf of patients who, on their own, do not select primary care physicians).

Target Oversight on Problem Providers

In time, the MCO learns which physicians consistently provide inappropriate services, engage in "creative" billing practices, or demonstrate patterns of substandard clinical practice. An MCO should target its oversight on problem physicians who are selected through objective, defensible, and uniformly applied criteria. Targeting enables MCOs to reduce the cost of some of their medical management programs and ease the burden on well-performing physicians.

Justify Programmatic Differences

In markets where physicians contract with many plans, they view the programmatic differences among MCOs as burdensome. As suggested earlier, that view conflicts with the health plans' need to innovate and to differentiate themselves in the market. Ideally, such innovations are viewed positively (not resented) by physicians. Regardless, an MCO should be up-front about its innovations—to patients and providers alike. It must clearly articulate to physicians the rationale for policy differences and how to comply with a policy's programmatic requirements. In addition, MCOs should not shrink from implementing programs and providing explanations that are based on customer preferences and demands.

Partner with Competitors

In programmatic areas that improve quality and/or relieve the administrative burden on physician practices, MCOs can work cooperatively, even with their competitors. Some functions that lend themselves to collaboration—and when performed properly should pass antitrust scrutiny—are credentials information collection, practice guideline development, and educational programs (e.g., academic detailing).

Provide Tangible Value

MCOs can provide measurable value to both physicians and their practices. For example, MCOs are better positioned than physicians to:

- develop and conduct multidisciplinary disease management programs which, at their core, enable physicians to provide higher quality patient care at a lower cost;

- mount prevention programs, especially for those healthy subscribers who do not visit their doctors very often; and

- provide physicians with feedback about their performance, particularly in comparison with peers—input that is highly valued.

Reward Positive Performance

Too many MCOs are viewed by physicians as concerned only about cost containment. Plans should offer financial rewards for non-cost-related performance, especially for activities related to the appropriate customer orientation of managed care. MCOs should consider awards for the availability of expanded office hours, higher patient satisfaction as measured by surveys and re-enrollment rates, and the attention paid to the provision of preventive care.

Involve Physicians

MCOs should give selected, interested physicians a meaningful role on committees, not waste their time with token participation. Also, MCOs should include physicians and other clinicians in management roles. Given the typically vast differences in backgrounds, skills, cultures, and goals of physicians and managed care administrators, the inclusion of physicians in senior management is one approach to barrier removal. Logically, physicians perform medical director-type functions, but these should not be the limit of their involvement. It is useful to include other informed physician viewpoints in most business activities, to help break down the cultural barriers described earlier.

Discipline Selectively and Wisely

Clear explanations about the nature of the problem and expectations for improvement are necessary with any physician who deviates significantly or consistently from key MCO requirements. It is advisable to terminate a refractory physician from the network without undue delay. No one, including the physician, gains from ongoing, adversarial relationships between a plan and a physician. However, caution is necessary when disciplining a physician with quality problems. In response to the public's interest in protection from incompetent physicians, the Health Care Quality Improvement Act of 1986 legislated a series of specific requirements to handle quality problems that include reporting requirements and due process for the involved physician.

■ Emerging Three-Tier Systems

The above steps apply to the interaction between health plans and physicians in the common open-panel, two-tier relationship. Given the inherent power gap between a health plan and a solo or small group practice, it is not surprising to find physicians aggregating their practices primarily to increase their contract negotiating power and to gain better leverage for themselves. Nevertheless, some physicians understand that, even in the face of a significant national backlash against managed care, market forces demand persistent attention to health care costs.

Newer forms of provider-based organizations—the capitated medical groups and new style IPAs on the West Coast, and the integrated delivery systems (IDS) that often include hospitals throughout the country—assume financial risk initially through their contracts with MCOs. These providers are organized intermediaries that perform many necessary managed care activities delegated by the MCO, including credentialing and utilization review activities.[69] (In this endeavor, the medical group, IPA, or IDS may actually purchase administrative services from a physician practice management company or medical service organization.)

In areas other than the West Coast, few at-risk provider organizations have been successful. Understandably, MCOs are reluctant to turn over their management responsibilities and capitated dollars to untested provider groups. The 1997 Balanced Budget Act permits provider-sponsored organizations (PSOs) to contract directly with Medicare on a capitated basis for beneficiaries who select care in the PSO under the new Medicare+Choice program. In a few places, such as Minneapolis, some employers bypass contracts with an MCO and instead contract directly with a provider organization.

The degree of success enjoyed by PSOs and similar organizations in direct contracting with payers is unclear. No one knows if these provider-based organizations can manage risk on subcontract to MCOs (echoing the dominant contracting model in California). For this model to succeed nationally, each organization must merge the physicians' attributes of professionalism with the values and orientation embedded in managed care. Whether individual professionals who value autonomy are able to accept the discipline required to compete on a cost basis in a marketplace environment remains to be seen. Nevertheless, the best chance to reshape health delivery by incorporating the strongest attributes of both professionalism and managed care may come from those provider organizations with the requisite capital and leadership to forge new entities.

■ Conclusion

Until now, the expansion in managed care has occurred primarily in IPA-model HMOs, PPOs, and point-of-service (POS) plans that offer consumers a broad choice of physicians. Although responsive to patient desires, this trend toward broader networks makes the MCO task of managing care more difficult. Yet even in today's environment, plans that work in collaboration with physicians may ultimately experience a market advantage, particularly as employers seek more value in their purchases of health insurance products. In contrast, the marketplace is impelling physicians and others to form organizations that can manage financial risk and assume some of the typical activities currently performed by MCOs. MCOs need to decide if they want to resist these efforts by organized provider groups or, alternatively, to join them.

■ Key Terms

Academic health centers (AHCs)
Core attitudes
Coverage exclusions
Different orientations
"Free-riders"

Market-driven arrangements
Partner with competitors
Physician buy-in
Reward positive performance

Risk selection
Tangible value
Target oversight
Three-tier system
Two-tier system
Values contrasts

Chapter 14

MEASURING AND MANAGING THE QUALITY OF CARE

■ Introduction

Traditionally, health insurance functions as a payer of claims, with little oversight over the type, frequency, or setting of services rendered, as long as the provider and facility are properly licensed. In contrast, an MCO also pays claims but it has much to say about what, how, when, by whom, and where services are rendered. This difference, reflected in the word "managed" in managed care, requires the MCO to monitor, scrutinize, approve, deny, or modify the process of care. In another contrast, traditional insurance typically pays for services by any licensed provider, while MCOs establish networks to better manage quality and costs. In yet another difference, MCOs may actively promote preventive services, such as mammograms and Pap smears, educate members about self-care, and provide information about how to use their system. A traditional health insurance company usually does not attempt to manage these quality-of-care-related functions or to measure results other than financial performance.

As MCOs succeeded in cost containment, a new vocabulary emerged to measure and report their success. Terms such as "bed days per thousand," "referrals per thousand," and "medical loss ratio" became the vernacular of the earliest and most prevalent form of control over health care: utilization management (UM). Physicians, hospital managers, Wall Street, and the general public learned about managed care through the language of UM. This created an impression of managed care as a system devoted to cost containment that places limits on choice of doctors and restricts access to health care services.

In comparison with hard utilization and financial metrics, early measures of quality of care and service for large populations were rudimentary and lacked clear definitions and the support of sophisticated computerized databases. Within the industry, MCOs and providers spent extensive time debating among peers about the many nuances related to measurement. They rarely spoke directly to the media or the general public about quality, a complicated topic that both groups fail to intuitively understand. This reticence resulted in a failure to communicate the basic message to consumers: Patients are better off when care is coordinated through a common venue and when the providers of care can communicate well about their care. Purchasers never understood (and most still don't) the nuances of MCO quality elements. Most were simply happy to know that an HMO was accredited or "federally qualified."

These deficiencies contributed to the industry's initial inability to explain the benefits and achievements of managed care to the American public. Attempts by the industry to talk to the media did not produce front-page copy to counter-point the prominence given to the "horror stories." The absence of a strong quality story during the early stages of managed care fueled the perception that quality was decidedly not the leading banner of a managed care organization. Today this impression remains, and is hard to shake.

■ Dual Role: Guardians of Cost and Quality

A significant challenge for MCOs is the maintenance of a credible balance between cost containment and quality. This challenge is complicated by a number of factors, including the following:

■ The public has long held the belief that more care, newer technology, and specialists constitute the best quality health care. Under fee-for-service, the proliferation of new technologies, procedures, drugs, etc. enjoyed almost unquestioned financial support. Easily found literature attests to the quality and/or effectiveness of a wide variety of contrasting and often competing diagnostic and therapeutic modalities. Thus, the best and most rigorously demonstrated clinical practices must compete with less well-demonstrated modalities for acceptance.

■ Two traditional guardians of quality, medical ethics and fear of litigation, are also cost-drivers. As viewed by most practitioners, the legal exposure occasioned by a reduction or withholding of certain health services outweighs the dangers of continuing to dispense excessive tests and treatments. The widespread proliferation of "defensive medicine" to preempt possible litigious action adds unnecessary layers of cost.

■ Academic medicine, the pharmaceutical industry, and medical device manufacturers are able to prove the effectiveness of treatments with new and costlier drugs and diagnostic tests. This ability results in the submission to and eventual approval by the Food and Drug Administration (FDA) of hundreds of new products. The FDA Modernization Act of 1997 facilitated the introduction of new products into the market. By contrast, demonstrating that old or existing treatments do not work—or that only marginal benefits are gained in comparison to less-costly existing technologies—is much less common because the required studies are large and expensive, do not support business growth, and are not academic career-builders.

■ The business of the health insurance industry is driven by a claims engine that is not equipped to factor in evidence-based appropriateness of care (e.g., the built-in claim "edits" that block payment for certain therapies).

These factors result in wide variations in care which, from a marketplace perspective, are understandable but costly. After reducing costs through contract negotiations with providers and limiting access to unproven resources, MCOs still face a difficult task: how to manage and improve care, control costs, and change member and provider perceptions within a well-entrenched, defensive approach to practicing medicine.

■ Quality Is Important

In the prepaid model of an HMO, the better the health of its members, the less expensive their care. From this point of view, managed care is good business if it focuses on prevention and early detection because healthier populations can result in lower medical costs. In contrast, the first wave of cost containment by HMOs (in which payments did not decrease but the rate of increase was set at lower levels that were in line with the general inflation rate) was achieved by aggressive contracting with physicians and hospitals and by utilization management. This is one of the most direct aspects of pure financial cost control. By contrast, managing care closely relates to improving the quality of medical care and controlling costs, as shown by the following examples:

■ Treatment for a member with diabetes whose disease is well controlled may cost half as much as the care for a patient whose disease is poorly controlled.

■ Care for a patient with early-stage colon cancer costs considerably less than care for someone with metastatic disease at the time of diagnosis.

- Cost for the care of members who engage in risky behaviors such as smoking, not exercising, and not wearing seat belts is generally higher than for those with healthy lifestyles.

- Measures taken to prevent a single premature birth may save $50,000 for that claim.

Management of health risks for future diseases makes sense, especially if an HMO anticipates high levels of member retention. However, with a turnover rate in managed care averaging 20–30 percent per year, why would an HMO invest in prevention? There are at least three valid reasons:

1. As illustrated above, prevention or early detection of many illnesses or medical events is dramatically cost-effective over a relatively short time period.

2. The National Committee for Quality Assurance (NCQA) standards incorporate selected goals from the U.S. Public Health Service's "Healthy People 2000" as prevention-related quality benchmarks for HMOs. Consumers judge HMO quality of care by examining the results attained according to these standards.

3. As new enrollees receive their care through managed care (assuming one company's disenrollment represents another's new enrollees), they contribute to a positive cycle, one that results in a higher level of preventive measures. This benefits society at large, along with the HMO.

Ultimately, employers and individual consumers share the cost of health care premiums. Thus, it follows that the healthier the population in general, the lower the premiums, and that better control of medical costs benefits the economy by contributing to a lower rate of inflation. For an employer, a healthier work force reduces the cost for sick time and injuries and results in lower premiums.

An MCO must update its standards and employ a more sophisticated approach to quality if it is to prove its value and to overcome the difficulties described above. To achieve cost control and to produce expected profits, a paradigm shift must occur within MCO operations. MCO leaders must endorse the concept of health management and then act: They must allocate the resources and implement the policies necessary to measure and manage health and disease among their members. Their ability to accomplish this shift is aided by a number of innovations and technical advancements, including:

- affordable and powerful information management technologies;

- improved patient-based survey instruments;

- wide acceptance of the application of statistical methods to vast data sets to draw valid conclusions;

■ mass communication capabilities;

■ proliferation of clinical practice guidelines; and

■ a conceptual understanding of small-area variation analysis.

These advances give MCOs the tools necessary to create a system to cost-effectively manage care for populations of patients with similar medical problems.

■ Quality Does Vary

Despite professed conscientious and ethical clinical practices by individual physicians, significant variations exist in the care of patients with particular disorders. John Wennberg, M.D., at Dartmouth College, discovered the existence of large variations in the utilization of health services within small geographic areas—one of the most significant contributions to understanding health care delivery in the United States. For example, the 1997 *Dartmouth Atlas* reports that the number of days Medicare patients spent in the hospital in the last six months of life ranged from 4.4 days in some regions to 22.9 in others. It is unlikely that disease severity alone accounts for this five-fold difference. These variations relate more to factors such as the number of specialists in the area, rather than to differences in the needs of patients based on disease severity or prevalence.

Using population-based geographic analysis of claims data, MCOs can confirm a significant variance in health care resource utilization for the same condition in different geographic locations. The common first response of physicians who practice in areas with significant variance is to attribute the differences in practice patterns to the complexity of patients' illnesses. The so-called "My patients are sicker" claim is slowly changing as case-mix and severity-adjusted comparisons of practice patterns negate the argument.

After controlling for differences in demographic profiles and unit cost, the basic question that MCOs try to answer is, what is the right level of resource utilization for a specific disease or diagnosis? An answer can be approximated by applying the components of "best practice" espoused by reputable, evidence-based clinical practice guidelines. When the Health Care Financing Administration (HCFA) introduced its Prospective Payment System in 1983, MCOs and other groups at financial risk for managing the care of large populations adopted the use of clinical practice guidelines or best practices to reduce unnecessary variations in care. The gradual elimination of unproven practices through practice guidelines became a safe harbor for the dual role of cost containment and quality improvement. However, implementation of such guidelines has been a very difficult task.

171

Managing the quality and cost of care in this fashion is only possible because of the vast capacity of computers, which gives epidemiologists, statisticians, and physicians versed in "population-health" principles the ability to manipulate huge data sets. Advances in computer technology and user friendliness allow MCOs to manipulate large data sets, such as medical and pharmacy claims, and gain insight about patterns in resource utilization. Data can be easily sliced into the following categories, individually and in combination:

- HMO;
- employer group;
- geographic area;
- insurance product type (fully insured, self-insured, experience-rated);
- setting (inpatient, outpatient, emergency room); and
- provider type (primary care physician [PCP], specialist, chiropractor).

Under the fee-for-service system, actuarial models could partially predict total future cost. For example, an actuarial prediction of a 12 percent increase in medical cost prompted a proportional increase in premiums. It did not matter what diseases, surgical procedures, new technologies, or new drugs accounted for the observed phenomenon because traditional insurance companies lacked the mandate and infrastructure to influence or manage these variables. Under managed care, health care transactions by enrollees that result in claims or "encounters" provide the data substrate. MCOs can analyze results to make projections about future resource consumption. For example, statistical models of previous utilization patterns based on medical claims and pharmacy data are now used to predict disease-specific future health care utilization.

■ Quality Can Be Measured

The maxim that "If you can't measure it, it didn't happen" is as true for the health care industry as it is for manufacturing and other service industries. Competition in a free market requires evidence or proof of the value of the product sold. That places a premium on an MCO's ability to demonstrate results in financial terms and in service, medical care quality, and member satisfaction. MCOs have tried in several ways to manifest an interest in quality, including:

Accreditation

As employers gradually shifted their employees from fee-for-service to managed care, the most important measure of quality was accreditation. Lacking a well-developed conceptual framework and tools to measure quality, HMOs relied on accreditation as a stand-in. The need to assure purchasers that quality is stringently monitored caused HMOs to seek accreditation by the NCQA, or more recently, the Joint Commission on Accreditation of Healthcare Organizations (JCAHO), whose main focus is accreditation of hospitals and other health care facilities. Among the many items these agencies survey, they seek demonstrable evidence that members

■ are given adequate access to care;

■ are informed of their rights and responsibilities;

■ are not subjected to under-treatment; and

■ receive care from properly credentialed providers.

Quality Indicators

Employers accepted accreditation as a signal of quality, although employees remained relatively uninformed of its significance. When more employees transitioned to managed care, quality scrutiny shifted toward measures that offer more meaning to the consumer than does the approval stamp of accreditation. Scorecards were created to compare health plans on quality indicators. For example, NCQA's "report card," the *Health Plan Employer Data and Information Set* (HEDIS), compares plans using standard measures. Among the most visible sets of HEDIS measures are preventive services, such as childhood immunizations, and early detection programs, such as mammography for breast cancer and Pap smears for cervical cancer. These are important measures because they emphasize prevention, a basic quality tenet of care management.

TQM/CQI

Without a common, industrywide measurement system, health care managers borrowed from the manufacturing sector the ideas and principles of total quality management and continuous quality improvement. TQM/CQI concepts permeated MCOs, and the health care system in general, at a whirlwind pace. Doctors noticed the alarming rate at which non-clinicians applied these unfamiliar concepts across hospitals, group practices, and nursing homes. The pace was fueled primarily by the need to curtail costs and secondarily by the mandates imposed by accrediting agencies that incorporated TQM/CQI principles into their standards.

Unfortunately, these quality-related efforts were insufficient to demonstrate or improve quality or contain costs. Accreditation is expensive and is often criticized for its focus on processes and structures of care, instead of actual health outcomes across a population or for a disease or treatment. The use of quality indicators as a tool to standardize and improve medical practices has yet to become routine in MCO operations. TQM/CQI principles, when applied to health care, cannot fully realize their potential because, unlike a manufacturer, the MCO does not completely control all of its "raw materials" (i.e., patient compliance, provider training, and education) or control the entire "production" process (i.e., timely diagnosis and treatment).

MCOs must use key tools, such as variation analysis, and newer methods that include:

Evidence-based Medicine

Evidence-based medicine is the systematic selection of clinical processes that are based on well-designed studies. There is an accepted hierarchy of study design that offers the greatest degree of confidence in its conclusions.

1. Controlled experiments, which follow a set of patients who have been randomized into at least one group that receives an intervention and another group that does not, are considered to be the most rigorous study design and are likely to produce the most defensible results. In many drug trials, patients who have been randomized into the non-intervention group receive a placebo. Even the clinicians participating in the study do not know which patients receive the experimental drug and which receive the placebo.

2. When randomized trials are not available, studies that use a variety of so-called quasi-experimental designs are considered to be the next most rigorous study design. Cohort studies and case-control studies are examples.

3. Only in the absence of the above studies can "expert opinion" or anecdotal reports of observed clinical phenomena suggest what constitutes a best practice.

4. The least rigorous method is a case series. For example, a case series study would track clinical outcomes for a group of patients with a given disease, accompanied by descriptions of the treatments given (but lacking controls of any type). These studies are useful to generate new ideas and hypotheses about a specific disease or treatment, but should not be considered conclusive.

The best body of information from a search of evidence-based medicine is usually compiled into practice guidelines. These guidelines discourage wasteful tests and treatments and encourage proven ones. The emerging, empirical evidence supports practice guidelines as a means to decrease medical costs while maintaining or improving health care quality.

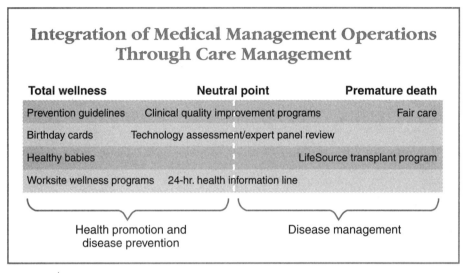

Figure 14.1

SOURCE: CIGNA HealthCare, Inc.

Patient-Centered Outcomes Measurement Instruments

The application of a consumer-centered perspective to the measurement of outcomes of care has created a number of scientifically designed and validated questionnaires or instruments (see below). These assessment tools capture the patients' perspectives about their general health or about their care for specific diseases. The results may differ significantly from their physicians' perspectives, even when treatment results in the desired outcome.

■ Quality Can Be Improved

Before the medical needs of aging baby boomers (just now entering their mid-50s) escalate demands on the health care system, MCOs must attend to measuring, improving, and maintaining the health status of their entire population along the continuum of care. More than 50 percent of medical problems are estimated to relate to lifestyle rather than genetic, environmental, or other external factors. Therefore, it seems logical that MCOs should commit sufficient resources to health promotion and disease prevention.

The health continuum model pictured in Figure 14.1 illustrates how an MCO designs programs to better manage all facets of an individual's total health care needs.

175

■ Managing Health

Managing health and managing diseases require that an MCO restructure its business. To manage health, MCOs begin with an assessment of members' health risks.

Assessment Tools

Assessment tools help gather information about measures to prevent diseases, called primary prevention (e.g., immunizations against polio). Complications or repeat episodes of an existing disease are labeled secondary prevention (e.g., giving baby aspirins to heart attack victims to prevent a subsequent heart attack). To assess health and health risks, an MCO obtains certain types of information directly from its members rather than from claims analysis. Three examples of assessments are:

1. Health Risks Assessments (HRAs)
   An MCO can use several voluntary survey instruments to ask adult members about health-related lifestyles such as tobacco use, seat belt use, and dietary habits. The survey may contain questions about the degree of readiness to change lifestyles and personal preferences for particular activities that reduce health risks. Typically, members receive a confidential, personal report that categorizes their most important risk factors, offers advice on how to decrease those risks, and occasionally recommends resources to aid in realizing those changes. Companies offering managed care plans to their employees are interested in the HRA results because risk factors are directly correlated with claims incurred by employees and dependents.

2. Quality of Life and Functional Status Assessments
   These questionnaires, designed to capture information about health-related quality of life, are divided into general health and disease-specific categories. Of these, the best known is the Short Form 36 Health Survey developed by John Ware. This type of questionnaire captures information about eight aspects of health:

   - physical functioning;
   - role-physical (ability to function in whatever role—parent, laborer, child of school age, etc.—without physical impediments);
   - bodily pain;
   - general health;
   - vitality;
   - social functioning;

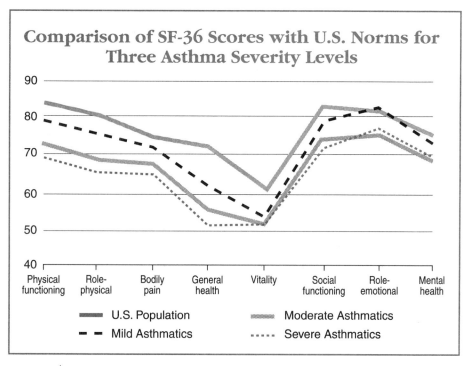

Figure 14.2

SOURCE: ITG Schering.

■ role-emotional (ability to function in society without emotional impediments); and

■ mental health.

For example, Figure 14.2 shows health profiles for U.S. adults with three levels of asthma severity, compared with U.S. norms.

3. Disease-Specific Questionnaires

These questionnaires focus on factors likely to be affected by the particular disease. For example, a depression-specific questionnaire asks about energy level, motivation, and self-esteem, whereas an instrument for low back pain queries the patient's pain levels and ability to climb stairs and lift objects. Many of these questionnaires are tested rigorously for their reliability and consistency. NCQA has already incorporated consumer satisfaction measures in HEDIS and has gone a step further by merging its Member Satisfaction Survey (MSS) with the Consumer Assessment of Health Plans Survey (CAHPS) for 1999 HEDIS reporting requirements. CAHPS focuses much more on reports of patients' experiences with health plans than on ratings of satisfaction.

Interventions

In addition to assessments of members' health, MCOs must offer intervention strategies to prevent disease and manage health. These include wellness programs and methods for early disease detection.

1. Wellness Programs

   Companies may offer wellness programs to their employees based on information obtained from HRAs and/or health care claim analysis. Employer-sponsored wellness programs are particularly attractive to self-insured employers in a managed care program because the economic benefits of a healthy employee population impact on productivity and decrease direct medical costs. Managed care organizations also sponsor wellness programs, typically in coordination with employers.

   Prevention and early detection programs are primarily the responsibility of MCOs working with contracted providers. Increasingly, employers sponsor worksite early detection programs such as mobile mammography units or on-site sigmoidoscopies for the early detection of colorectal cancer. Wellness programs may be structured as:

   ■ Promotional/educational

   This approach usually requires a dedicated staff and significant resources to reach the entire employee (and sometimes dependent) population. Participation in the programs is voluntary; there is no penalty for non-participation.

   ■ Incentive-based

   Incentive-based programs implemented by employers are enticing or coercive, depending on the dollar amounts forfeited by non-participants. Some incentive-based programs calculate premium differentials based on the results achieved because of participation in health promotion/disease prevention programs. For example, the company might establish premium differentials for employees who quit smoking, lose weight, or maintain good control of blood pressure. Figure 14.3 shows a graphic representation of a wellness and prevention program.

2. Prevention Programs

   Other MCO interventions relate to disease prevention, not to lifestyle. For example, immunization programs are proven effective independent of lifestyle. Prevention programs may also be combined with wellness programs (e.g.,

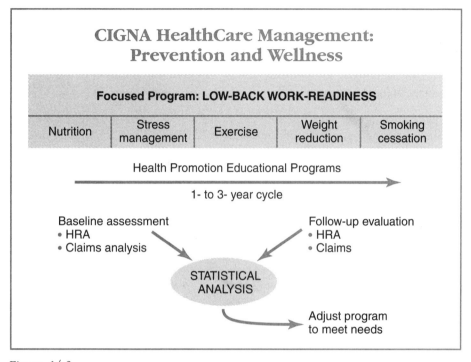

Figure 14.3

SOURCE: CIGNA HealthCare, Inc.

when hormone replacement therapy for post-menopausal women to prevent osteoporosis is combined with lifestyle adjustments such as exercise, smoking cessation, and adequate calcium intake in the diet).

3. Early Detection

The purpose of this intervention is to diagnose disease early in its natural history—even before symptoms are manifest. Examples of such interventions include mammography for early detection of breast cancer and Pap smears for cervical cancer.

Reporting Tools

Communicating the results of activities devoted to managing health is often referred to as an exercise in reporting "non-events." The only way to report these "non-events" is through a comparison of:

179

CIGNA HealthCare Mid-Atlantic: Study At-a-Glance

Study
Mammography screening

Primary objective
Improve compliance rate with mammography
screening guideline for women 50-64 years
during two-year period ending in reporting year

Measurement
HEDIS administrative methodology

Interventions
Birthday card reminder
Articles in *Well Being*

Performance goal
Health plan 1995 = 70%
Health plan year 2000 = 80%
Healthy people 2000 = 60%

1994-1995 Results
Percentage of Women
Having Screening

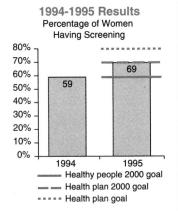

Healthy people 2000 goal
Health plan 2000 goal
Health plan goal

Planned Improvements: Birthday card, newsletters, letters to non-compliant women

Figure 14.4

SOURCE: CIGNA HealthCare, Inc.

■ current events against previous period events in like populations; or

■ age-sex and severity-adjusted controls, ideally within the same company.

Often such comparisons are not possible because the MCO lacks complete
data. MCOs must overcome this obstacle and design methods to report "non-
events" as a benefit to both providers and members. CIGNA's *Study At-a-
Glance* (Figure 14.4) demonstrates one format for information reporting.

■ Managing Disease

MCOs are prime customers for disease management programs because of their
ability to analyze claims data and identify populations of members with specific
conditions. Disease management offers a logical approach to improving quality
of care because it

■ leverages the innovations identified above to improve health outcomes;

■ fosters more efficient processes;

CIGNA HealthCare Priorities for Care Management

Disease	Costly?	Frequent?	Changeable?	Feasible?	Measurable?	Total

Assign each cell a score from 1-5 and add up the total. You can introduce a greater level of "precision" if you weigh each column differently depending on your priorities and multiply the score by the weighing factor and then total it.

Figure 14.5

SOURCE: CIGNA HealthCare, Inc.

■ maintains or improves disease-related quality of life (and its functional status enhances patient and provider satisfaction); and

■ lowers health care costs.

Development of a Disease Management Program

MCOs that choose to implement disease management begin the process by applying a population-based approach, using the epidemiological methods of the public health sector to set priorities for health improvement. First, the organization determines priorities among many clinical entities by using a predefined set of criteria. The matrix used by CIGNA HealthCare is shown in Figure 14.5. It asks five questions: Is the condition frequent, costly, changeable, and measurable, and is it feasible for the company to execute the program?

Components of a Disease Management Program

Disease management programs may be comprehensive and complex or simple and focused. The definition of precise, measurable objectives dictates the program's scope, depth, and budget, helps define both the interventions and the metrics necessary to measure results, and identifies personnel who should par-

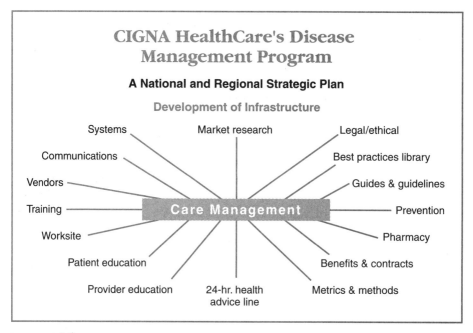

CIGNA HealthCare's Disease Management Program

A National and Regional Strategic Plan

Development of Infrastructure

Systems · Market research · Legal/ethical

Communications · Best practices library

Vendors · Guides & guidelines

Training — Care Management — Prevention

Worksite · Pharmacy

Patient education · Benefits & contracts

Provider education · 24-hr. health advice line · Metrics & methods

Figure 14.6

SOURCE: CIGNA HealthCare, Inc.

ticipate. For example, CIGNA HealthCare's diabetes disease management program calls for a highly complex support structure that involves:

1. Confirmation (after members are identified) of the diagnosis through a telephone interview. The patient's primary care physician is notified of the patient's eligibility for educational interventions to help manage his or her condition, according to doctor's instructions.

2. Employers, whether self-insured or fully insured, are notified that the program is in effect (without revealing any employee's identity).

3. A team of lawyers and ethicists oversees issues that relate to patient confidentiality and ensures that risk management concerns are addressed.

4. Another team of information management and systems experts supports all aspects of data collection, storage, processing, and reporting.

5. Medical teams oversee the specific contents of the patient-member educational program to ensure that appropriate guidelines are followed (in the case of diabetes, the American Diabetes Association's standards of care).

6. A "complex" disease management program also has a mechanism for reviewing and updating the contents of the program over time, based on new knowledge from the medical literature or "lessons learned" from the implementation process itself.

A schematic representation of CIGNA HealthCare's disease management program is shown in Figure 14.6.

Defining Intervention Modalities

Interventions usually match disease severity, as established by explicit stratification criteria. In the diabetes example, the results of the Hemoglobin A1c blood test is an ideal clinical element to stratify disease severity. In the absence of clinical data, resource utilization is a surrogate indicator. The tables below demonstrate a typical stratification method and show how the sickest members receive greater attention.

Data Management

An MCO's claims database serves as a source to identify disease prevalence among its population. For example, a recent review at CIGNA HealthCare of the distribution of health care costs by ICD–9 major diagnostic categories reveals the three top claim categories as musculoskeletal disorders, cardiovascular disorders, and cancers. Within each category, the specific diseases that account for a significant proportion of the claims are targets for disease management programs.

Table 14.1

Sample Stratification Method

	Member stratification criteria			
Definitive	**Level I**	**Level II**	**Level III**	**Level IV**
Hemoglobin Alc	<8%	8%–10%	10%–12%	>12%
Interim stratification	**Level I**	**Level II**	**Level III**	**Level IV**
Primary diabetes— admission or ER claim past 12 months	No	1	2	3 or more
Insulin using	No	Yes	N/A	N/A

SOURCE: Copyright, Diabetes Treatment Center of America, Inc. Used by permission.

Table 14.2

A Sample Intervention Plan

WellAware℠ for Diabetes Member interventions Level II, III, IV	
Activity	**Frequency**
Metabolic management assessment (telephonic)	One time
Diabetes goal plan	Initial with quarterly updates
Diabetes care calls	
Level II	Every 6 weeks
Level III	Monthly
Level IV	Bi-weekly
Diabetes education communications	As needed

SOURCE: Copyright, Diabetes Treatment Center of America, Inc. Used by permission.

Data Availability

Disease management programs are feasible only to the extent that data in sufficient quantity and quality are available. The best disease management programs usually rely on data that can be integrated, such as claims, encounters, pharmacy, eligibility, provider files, health risk assessment, home health, etc. The databases must share common fields (e.g., patient identifiers) to link a member with the right provider to the right prescription. A common predicament occurs when data are unavailable, usually for two reasons:

1. Under capitation, providers lack an incentive to submit encounter records—the equivalent to claim records—for services rendered. Because providers receive pre-payments or capitation for patients' care, submission of encounter records is an administrative burden not essential to payment collection. However, the absence of encounter data produces information gaps that significantly affect an MCO's ability to identify members for disease management activity. MCOs must devote a significant amount of time and effort to the collection of encounter data.

2. Another gap occurs when an employer carves out services and the MCO is unable to access the claims data. For example, when pharmacy benefits are carved out, the MCO may be unable to query a prescriptions database for insulin to identify its members with diabetes. To overcome this, the MCO must import pharmacy data from the carve-out vendor, or the pharmacy vendor (frequently a pharmacy benefit management company) imports the pertinent claims data to identify potential members for the disease management intervention.

Identification of the required data, an understanding of their use, and a determination of their availability are all essential to assess the objectives of a disease management program. The five categories subject to measurement are:

- Processes of care: Was a test done?

- Outcomes of care: What was the test result? Is it normal?

- Quality of life and functional status: As a result of treatment, is the member better able to function on a day-to-day basis?

- Satisfaction with medical care and service.

- Cost of care.

Data Analysis

The data and analysis must be sound so that resources to manage disease states can be allocated properly. For example, determining the cost-effectiveness of a diabetes disease management program requires the measurement of all medical costs before and after implementation to determine the following:

- Are observed changes due strictly to the program?

- Do confounding variables exist, such as a new contract with a hospital that lowers hospitalization costs for all members regardless of diagnosis?

- Did the group of members enrolled in the program represent the very sickest?

- Is any re-measurement of the cost of care likely to produce lower numbers, even without any intervention, because of the law of regression toward the mean?

- Are comparisons of the cost-effectiveness of a program offered at two or more locations truly valid?

- Is there assurance that sicker patients are not concentrated in one location, perhaps because of the presence of a very competent specialist physician?

These and many other variables may hide the true impact of a disease management program. Thus, strong statistical support is mandatory, preferably early in the planning stages. Statistical measures sometimes control for some confounding variables, but more important, they help establish the confidence level in the conclusions reached during the analysis of outcomes.

Confidentiality

Confidentiality is a primary concern in health care. It is particularly important when massive amounts of data are transferred electronically. Processes such as

185

security audits of vendors, passwords, locked facilities, restricting access to data only to essential personnel, encryption protocols, etc. are necessary to help protect the information. The future of data management includes the ability of MCOs to make member-specific information available online to providers directly, via the Internet or intranets. For example, an HMO may prepare, by physician panel, a list of women without recent mammograms whose first-degree relatives had breast cancer. As these women are considered a high-risk cohort for breast cancer, their physicians can encourage each to have a mammogram.

Reporting Results

Disease management programs need simple reporting formats. Often reports are read by non-clinicians and non-researchers. Presentation of the results in graphical representations is recommended; it is more intuitive and user-friendly than a spreadsheet filled with numbers. Another characteristic of a good disease management report is its usefulness to MCOs and their customers in making business decisions.

Paying for Health and Disease Management Programs

Many employers assume that health management and disease management programs are an integral part of the "package" they purchase from an MCO. Until recently, that was not the case. Disease management gained popularity as an added value service that would reduce medical costs and improve quality. The cost of administering these programs either has been incorporated into the rates quoted by the MCO or is charged separately. The charging mechanism is problematic, given contract terms with employers, physicians, and ancillary service providers (such as home health and laboratory). For example, an MCO's disease management program may not result in cost savings to the employer group if the physicians who care for those patients are capitated. Instead, savings accrue to the provider group. To turn the actual reductions in medical resource utilization by the disease management program into savings to employers, MCOs are limited to:

■ incorporating such savings into the calculations for subsequent-year contracts with providers; and

■ sharing the savings among employers, the MCO, and the providers, which, in turn, should result in lower or stable premiums to individuals.

Ethical and Medico-Legal Considerations

Disease management programs must receive close review and scrutiny by a competent lawyer and an ethicist. These programs often challenge conventional rules of engagement among doctors, MCOs, employers, pharmacy benefit management companies, and vendors working on behalf of the MCO.

Anticipating questions of ethics is an important consideration whenever an MCO introduces a new concept or program that (outside of managed care) may be controversial. For example, a program to address the issue of death with dignity and the avoidance of futile care under an HMO quickly may become a target of vituperative criticism based on an erroneous assumption that such a program is motivated by financial interests.

■ Conclusion

Under the prepaid covenant, MCOs assume responsibility for members' care, spanning the continuum of services from prevention through rehabilitation or control of chronic and terminal diseases. To achieve long-term economic survival, MCOs must gain control over the existing inefficiencies of caring for illnesses (especially chronic ones). In this mode, good medicine—and good business—is defined by how well an MCO maintains healthy members, diagnoses and treats conditions early, and fosters the use of evidence-based medicine. Health promotion and disease prevention are financially rewarded.

With a focus on health prevention and disease management, MCOs can better control the quality of medical care and its costs. These programs must become the competitive advantage for an MCO and, if effective, may help convince a skeptical public that their MCO is concerned about their health, not just their premiums. Optimally, the programs can reverse the public's negative perception of managed care—a perception so prevalent that advocacy groups, malpractice attorneys, the media, and legislators capitalize on it in their respective domains.

■ Key Terms

Accreditation	Consumer Assessment	Disease
Clinical practice	of Health Plans Survey	management
guidelines	(CAHPS)	Disease-specific
Confidentiality	Data management	questionnaires

Ethical, medico-legal considerations
Evidence-based medicine
FDA Modernization Act of 1997
Health continuum model
Health management
Health Plan Employer Data and Information Set (HEDIS)
Health risk assessments (HRAs)
Intervention modalities
Joint Commission on Accreditation of Healthcare Organizations (JCAHO)

National Committee for Quality Assurance (NCQA)
Patient-centered outcomes measurement
Population-based geographic analysis
Practice guidelines
Prevention programs
Primary prevention
Quality indicators
Quality of life and functional status assessment
Reporting results
Secondary prevention

Short Form 36 Health Survey
Small-area variation analysis
Total quality management/ continuous quality improvement (TQM/ CQI)
Utilization management (UM)
Wellness programs

Chapter 15

MANAGING MARKET-DRIVEN ORGANIZATIONAL CHANGE

■ Introduction

Price competition, capacity consolidation, and financial risk arrangements are powerful market forces influencing the restructuring of the entire health care industry. Few organizations escape these industry dynamics.

■ Physicians join larger medical groups or join physician practice management companies, and hospitals continue to merge or affiliate with each other and with other providers to form larger health systems. At a minimum, the market prompts more service integration between health plan administration and patient care delivery functions, among facilities and practitioners, and within institutions through comprehensive case management and individualized care protocols. The market's need for substantially lower health care premiums compels health providers to face the stark reality that industrywide consolidation will produce a few clear winners and many losers.

■ Purchasers demand more value from providers, elevating quality to a high priority. Perceived value (not just cost control) becomes a criterion from which to judge health care adequacy. Many MCOs and providers embraced continuous quality improvement principles, and a few can adequately demonstrate effective medical management, better treatment outcomes, and improved customer satisfaction. Value must be documented to earn purchasers' premiums and ongoing business trust.

■ Health care organizations cannot sufficiently reduce their operating costs without sustained efforts. Even short-term strategies such as consolidation (or reduced working capital) may lead to the rationing of access to services or an inability to replace fixed assets. Business as usual, even when improved (via incremental changes on a piecemeal basis) no longer suffices to address customer demands for significant cost reduction and improved service quality.

■ Since the early 1980s, MCOs have decreased costs through techniques such as preauthorization, case management, and negotiated discounts from fee schedules. MCOs exerted systematic cost controls on all providers: networks, physician specialists, hospitals, allied health professionals, and ancillary services vendors. Finally, to improve their financial performance, MCOs increased the financial risk for individual providers by implementing capitated or budget-based reimbursement.

As these market forces continue to define stringent cost and performance targets for health care organizations, reengineering methodologies become an essential survival tool to manage change and improve service. Premium rates can be incrementally reduced only so far before payment no longer covers real costs. Premiums can be increased only so much before payers look toward less expensive alternatives, such as direct contracting with providers for services.

This challenge for economic survival requires a tremendous cultural change—a different way of doing business—for everyone involved in the delivery and financing of health care. Critics claim that financial incentives that are too closely aligned pose a potential ethical challenge. How can the clinical practice of medicine (which formerly operated at arm's length from cost management) balance the patient's interest in access to appropriate health care services with the MCO's interests in economizing, maintaining profit margins, and producing satisfied customers? This is not an insurmountable challenge: The integration of provider and payer functions can create compensation and reward systems to serve both ends. However, the delivery system's business values must adhere to a philosophical commitment to four practices:

■ preventive care;

■ early detection and appropriate treatment of disease;

■ health promotion and education services; and

■ objective performance measures.

The incorporation of these practices forces provider networks or organizations to rethink what they do and how they do it. Their success depends on motivating employees, rewarding desired behavior, and reinforcing the need for organizational and individual change. A substantial change in direction compels both MCOs and providers to:

■ reexamine how health care services are structured;

■ critically assess how health care services are organized and delivered; and

■ consider whose needs are being served and what results are achieved.

■ Managing Delivery System Redesign

Keeping members healthy for as long as possible and targeting appropriate treatment goals for specific illnesses meet the needs of patients and support financial accountability. To accomplish these objectives, an MCO must reorganize crucial aspects of its business, including its relationships with stakeholders (providers, purchasers, and members). It must design a strategy for change that acknowledges the corporate culture within its own organization and the values of each stakeholder. Initiation of a reorganization effort is predicated on the establishment of key change principles:

Partnership with Stakeholders

An MCO should seek ways to align all of its stakeholders with its long-term strategic objectives. It must present a unifying theme (e.g., cost-effective, quality care) and a common frame of reference (e.g., fixed payment) to align different organizational strategies and financial incentives among business partners. The spotlight moves away from an organizational focus to a member or patient focus. Collaboration works better than adversarial competition if the process is thoughtfully managed. The creation of a true partnership among health plan members, health professionals, and MCOs requires stakeholders to:

- explicitly define their individual roles and responsibilities in relation to each other;
- foster new business relationships and interdependency by forcing aggressive patient management at each point along a continuum of care;
- identify shared business goals and a strategy to support the key values (e.g., quality care, customer service) of each stakeholder;
- gain the buy-in of providers, particularly physicians, through financial distribution formulas that are simple, easy to understand, and fair;
- require practitioners to accept accountability for compliance with the performance standards (e.g., productivity requirements, patient satisfaction measures, and quality indicators); and
- encourage (and assist) health care organizations to reengineer day-to-day clinical behavior and administrative procedures to create greater efficiency and effectiveness in keeping with mutually accepted goals and objectives.

Develop a Change Strategy

In any health care organization, there are numerous voices for change but little agreement on specifics or pace. Moreover, administrators, technical staff, physicians, and customers all have different perspectives on how an organization should change. Usually, constituents overwhelmingly support the maintenance of the status quo, because organizational change is disruptive and is often personally threatening to those involved.

Shared values and trust are the most important resources an organization draws on to reposition itself through reengineering. They are the basis for collaborative decision-making across all organizational levels and professional disciplines and are prerequisites for changing an organization's corporate culture. The organizational and personal turbulence often caused by transition must be acknowledged and factored into redesign strategies. Moreover, changes must be orchestrated and managed to reflect and maintain both shared values and trust. The process calls for leadership and change management skills not commonly found in organizations patterned on the command-and-control management style typical in health care institutions.

Recognize Corporate Cultures

Change must be presented as an expression of the organization's culture. For example, measuring improvement in member health status as an indicator of performance suggests large-scale organizational change, but not a change in values. A change of this magnitude demands a fully developed strategy to implement a new business model. A corporate cultural strategy is necessary to motivate physicians—often the individuals most likely to challenge reengineering efforts. Physician buy-in makes a significant contribution to the improvement of clinical efficiency, quality, and patient satisfaction.

The corporate culture of an organization, and the subcultures of its divisions and departments, must be examined for potential obstacles to reengineering activities. Health plans and other organizations often ignore corporate culture as a critical factor in the success of capitation, despite its pervasive influence. They regard corporate culture as a soft, nebulous notion that is neither readily defined nor translated into concrete management actions. In fact, mergers of companies have failed or never materialized because of incompatible corporate cultures. The cultural strategy connects the overall business strategy with the day-to-day operating and reimbursement strategies.

■ Reengineering the Organization

The reengineering process creates a particular momentum and direction, depending on how aggressively senior management pushes and on the extent of change an organization can withstand and manage. The need to reengineer and the parameters for how much and how fast organizations must change are also influenced by local marketplace forces.

■ Reengineering Is Not. . .
Typically, organizations experience lesser, incremental changes before recognizing that more fundamental, radical change is needed. An organization might start down the path of reengineering by analyzing how business is conducted. This analysis identifies problems and potential solutions that lead to the reworking of a particular function, product line, or organizational component. The analysis and redesign activity often results in changing work roles to reduce costs and improve productivity. Often labeled as reengineering, this activity is actually rightsizing or downsizing. Downsizing is not reengineering, nor is it a viable long-term business strategy because it does not increase revenue, create new products, or increase opportunities for growth.

■ Reengineering Is. . .
Reengineering represents a methodology for thinking about work, organizational purpose, and performance. It is a developmental and evolutionary process that follows a logical sequence of events, but rarely progresses in a linear manner. Successful reengineering emphasizes a few key ingredients: simplifying and redesigning how people work, improving their job skills, motivating them to perform better, and providing the necessary equipment, technology, and facility support. Reengineering is neither an answer nor an end in itself, but is a means to an end. Its success depends on an organization's commitment and ability to manage fundamental change.

Start with Key Questions

In their reengineering efforts, health care organizations of all types struggle to resolve these six fundamental business questions that determine their marketplace success or failure:

1. Which services does the organization perform alone, and which are performed in conjunction with others through virtual relationships or subcontracts?

2. How can services be performed according to a personal care plan for each member, one that projects health care needs throughout a member's life and serves as a frame of reference for episodic care?

3. What are the required services that (through restructured relationships within and among delivery systems) hospitals, subacute facilities, medical groups, and allied health professionals should address to reduce costs and improve clinical and service quality?

4. Who should perform a particular service, based on redesigned patient care teams—multidisciplinary, primary care-based—and self-care management guidelines and instructions?

5. Where should a service be performed, based on patient convenience, treatment efficacy, and availability of subacute services and settings?

6. How should provider compensation be structured in order to increase motivation and reward performance that meets patient needs, customer expectations, and organizational goals?

Answers to these questions lead to a programmatic reorientation from an organization/provider-based philosophy to a customer-driven philosophy. The reorientation calls for fundamental shifts in ideology, institutional priorities, and direction for the health care industry and embodies a change in values that affects everyone's daily roles and responsibilities. The questions are often viewed as a threat, because they force hospitals and physicians to reevaluate their services from a patient's point of view. Likewise, the process forces managed care organizations to judge their services from member and employer perspectives. Each role change represents a break from the previous "business as usual" approach.

Thus, one reengineering goal is to increase customer satisfaction through seamless delivery of care among different services and vendors. Making patient care and members' services truly seamless requires rethinking and redesigning the individual components of the current delivery system. Purchasers and plan members want fully integrated services across the continuum of care that are user-friendly and transparently coordinated. This challenge involves integrating each clinical discipline with each functional department, thereby replacing a traditional departmental approach with an interdisciplinary cross-departmental approach to patient care. The redesign plan must address both the clinical systems and the management and support systems that constitute an integrated health system.

Reengineer Management and Support Systems

When health care organizations are restructured based on reengineering principles (e.g., work redesign, customer focus, service integration, management restructuring, and cross training), their form and function change accordingly. For example:

■ Traditional organizational charts with lines and boxes are modified and complemented by role relationships that explain how individuals and business units must support each other in meeting customer service goals and financial targets. These new interrelationships stress partnership, accountability, and an explicit customer service orientation.

Table 15.1

Health Care Reengineering Phases

Phase one	Phase two	Phase three	Phase four
Analyze business: ■ problems ■ opportunities Redesign work roles Reduce costs	Restructure management Automate functions Redesign clinical services and standardize treatment protocols Align provider financial incentives: ■ physicians ■ other practitioners ■ hospitals ■ ancillary services	Develop a member focus Create personal care plans Integrate information components: ■ administrative ■ clinical ■ financial ■ member ■ demographic Standardize care for patient groups	Integrate clinical disciplines and functional departments Integrate core functions: ■ patient care delivery ■ health plan administration ■ community-based services

SOURCE: Boland: *Redesigning Healthcare Delivery*, Chapter 1, p. 10.

■ Senior management must support those frontline staff who have the most contact with customers (including physicians), and remove bureaucratic obstacles to help them better serve patients and members.

Once reengineered activities are implemented, the organization adapts, and the project enters a new phase of refinement. Other core business functions are then targeted for redesign, further expanding the circle of reengineering projects.

Ultimately, MCOs must configure service delivery to provide a full continuum of care for members. For many, this means assembling a "virtually" (rather than a vertically or horizontally) integrated company. Participants' assets are not necessarily merged. Instead, their service components are managed through contractual relationships. The virtual organizational approach implies a different structure and management orientation to care delivery, but it must remain centered on the improvement of members' health status.

Redesign Management

Senior management must lead reengineering efforts, often by first restructuring itself to gain credibility and to demonstrate its expertise. Management restructuring seeks to reduce the number of layers between top management, practitioners, and patients. Different points in the process may result in repeated

195

restructuring of each layer of management. Restructuring gives more responsibility and authority to individuals who have direct contact with patients and plan members. This leads to greater accountability, reduced cost, better service quality, and increased patient satisfaction. In addition, it is important to automate as many administrative functions as possible to increase efficiency and customer service.

Eliminate Redundant Activities

There is currently little emphasis on integrating and consolidating providers' and health plans' roles to reduce operating costs and improve service quality. Yet redundancy is a critical shortcoming of many delivery systems; if corrected, dramatic systemwide savings can occur. To eliminate redundancy, partnering organizations must relinquish certain administrative functions, even those that generate revenue. To accomplish this task, each overlapping activity is critically evaluated to determine:

- Should it be provided at all?
- If so, by whom and where should it be provided?
- Do competitive market forces compel the need for separate activities?
- Do regulatory, accreditation, or legal issues prevent the merger of—or require—separate activities?

For example, utilization management responsibilities and activities are often administered separately—and redundantly—by health plans, hospitals, medical groups, allied health practitioners, and numerous third-party vendors. MCOs, in an effort to distinguish themselves from competitors, sell purchasers on the effectiveness of their utilization review efforts. The MCO may be evaluated by accrediting agencies, in part, on its utilization review program. Providers must maintain their own utilization programs to control resource consumption and to meet requirements of payers, regulators, and surveyors (which may be different agencies with different rules or criteria). This example illustrates the complexity involved in changing a function that is redundant and costly, even when the change could streamline the administrative burden and costs for everyone.

Eventually, purchasers and payers want a significant level of cost removed from health care delivery and will select vendors that can do so. However, the question must be asked: Do most health plans or delivery systems have the organizational resources (in terms of capital, information technology, and management depth)—and the political will—to reduce overlapping functions? There is an emerging need for "system integrators" that can provide these resources for each market. The most likely candidates are technology companies, advanced

MANAGING MARKET-DRIVEN ORGANIZATIONAL CHANGE

provider organizations, and delivery systems with substantial capital access, or joint venture arrangements among these stakeholders.

Expand Staff Competence

Although technology helps drive change and is a prerequisite for successful re-engineering, the process is primarily about people. Staff skills, knowledge, and work roles must expand and integrate to meet customer needs.

Managing the human side of organizational change is now a major challenge faced by the health care industry. Ongoing training for employees is necessary if they are to acquire the skills that fit the new work responsibilities resulting from system reengineering efforts. Employees and employers must clearly understand their mutual responsibilities during each phase of reengineering and as a result of organizational restructuring. Otherwise, organizations ignore a key potential benefit of reengineering: learning faster than the competition. To be successful and profitable, health care organizations must demonstrate the critical linkage between human resources, organizational learning, and overall business strategy.

Involve Customers

MCOs must encourage and enable customers to assume more responsibility as partners to reduce the need for costly care and to improve medical outcomes. Employers may become involved in redesigning care delivery that uses a systems approach to reduce costs, improve quality, and increase customer satisfaction. At a minimum, employers can contribute more to benefits design, work site safety, and injury prevention. Their involvement can extend to include lifestyle risk management programs, employee incentives, and early screening and referral mechanisms, such as employee assistance programs. In 1998, there were only a few instances of established strategic partnerships. For most employers, health care is not a primary business; their main interest is to purchase medical benefits as cheaply as possible. This situation may change as employers look to increase benefits (with little additional cost) as a means to attract or retain employees in a competitive job market.

Focus on Core Competencies

Organizations require sufficient management depth, skills, and knowledge to be successful in an evolving market. Challenging institutional beliefs and assumptions is not enough: Organizations must know how to accomplish new tasks and redesign existing programs. Basic core competencies must exist in:

■ change management;

■ project management; and

■ customer management.

Employ New Technology and Comprehensive Information Systems

One of the most important factors in any re-design is the improvement that new technology makes possible, both in quality of care and in overall system performance. Significant technological advances permit the restructuring of health care by changing the setting in which services are appropriately provided, by training lesser-skilled individuals to perform services, and by reducing patients' recovery time and care. Technology regularly allows procedures and treatments to be safely performed in physicians' offices and other ambulatory settings that once required intense (and expensive) hospital services.

Advances in management information systems provide people and organizations with new and better ways to communicate, analyze data, structure organizations, and reduce the cost of doing business. Effective information systems are necessary to support fundamental tenets of managed care, such as continuity of services across the continuum of care and monitoring of financial performance.

A growing emphasis on accountability mandates that delivery systems consolidate most of their data repositories, information services, and reporting functions. This consolidation enables integration of administrative, clinical, and financial data into easy-to-understand and comprehensive reports. It helps meet the employers' need for more "actionable data" to make better decisions about designing employee benefits. Health plans need more flexible and focused information systems to manage provider networks and document the effect of their services on the health of enrollees.

Reengineer Clinical Care and Systems

If the overall goal is to better serve health plan members and patients, then an organization must also redesign its care-giving services around its members' health needs and cultural sensitivities. Redesign efforts that target clinical services sometimes begin with a continuous quality improvement program and standardized patient care protocols. Although this approach may marginally improve the clinical quality of care, it does not dramatically increase savings or service quality.

Health plans and providers that function under capitated arrangements may find it too costly to wait until a member is acutely ill or in need of chronic care services. More aggressive health care interventions may be called for. However, the amount of time required for most illness prevention services to make an impact in terms of reduced need for acute care services is not known. Meaningful cost savings and breakthroughs in member satisfaction require a rethinking of the full continuum of care and individual services. The necessary components for the successful redesign of clinical systems and care delivery include the following:

Establish Clinical Practice Guidelines

Clinical process reengineering emphasizes the development of standardized treatment protocols for specific types of patients. In combination with feedback from outcomes measurements and research, the most effective treatments become standardized clinical practice guidelines or protocols that are applied, when appropriate, to whole groups of patients.

Embrace Population-Based Disease Management

Managed care strategies must change the focus of health care activities from a single incidence of patient care to management of the care of all enrollees covered under a contract. "Population-based" care incorporates all the necessary services, practitioners, and treatment settings needed by health plan members. Disease management addresses groups of patients, not just individual episodes of illness. The objective is to better manage the health risk of target groups, which extend well beyond acute care patients and chronically ill members. Management emphasizes risk-driven (instead of event-driven) care, such as:

- use of preventive services to reduce the likelihood of illness;
- early detection and the use of screening services to intervene sooner in the illness cycle; and
- matching specific medical and social services to target groups.

Delivery systems must change if they are to intervene in illness sooner and more effectively. By influencing the underlying causes of controllable, acute care episodes (e.g., preventable accidents and injuries, and behaviorally linked illness), health plans realize financial savings and members develop and maintain better lifestyles.

Develop Personal Care Plans

One of reengineering's major challenges is the development of a strong member focus for all organizational activities. One component of this focus is the creation of personal care plans for all enrollees and their dependents. Personal

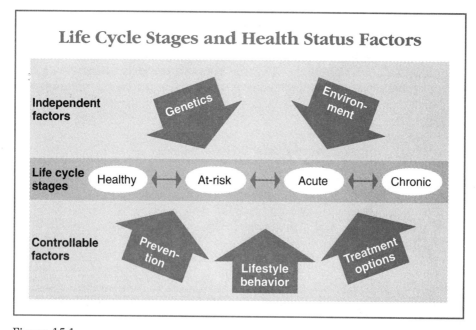

Life Cycle Stages and Health Status Factors

Figure 15.1

SOURCE: Boland: *Redesigning Healthcare Delivery,* Chapter 1, p. 20.

care plans address members' current and expected health care needs based on demographic characteristics and identifiable risk factors, including family history.

Monitor High-Risk, High-Cost Patients

As more risk is transferred from public payers and employers to health plans and providers, the latter must manage, under capitated payments, the care of high-risk, high-cost groups such as the frail elderly and chronically ill adults and children. Operating with a risk management focus, delivery systems can maximize their resources by monitoring their plan members' health status and patient functioning before allocating effective, appropriate services.

Managed Chronic Care

One of the most far-reaching economic and clinical challenges facing managed care is the growing demand for the management of chronic care conditions. Managed care delivery systems are deeply rooted in the acute care model. This model is not geared to managing care for an aging population that includes many patients with incurable chronic illness who need relief of symptoms and prevention of further dysfunction. Instead, a biopsychosocial model (i.e., medical, social, and community orientation) is required, one that encompasses more than the physiological factors commonly associated with acute care treatment. The goal of chronic care management is not curative; emphasis is on the improvement or maintenance of the quality of life and level of function. MCOs must find effective methods to provide chronic care through team-based care management, telemedicine, and other methods that can be far more cost-effective than the traditional physician-based, facility-centered treatment models.

Use Multidisciplinary Teams

For the chronic care population (i.e., high-cost/high-risk individuals), a multidisciplinary team approach integrates primary and specialty care with home-based and community-based services. The team integrates both patient and family perspectives into the care process, making treatment more effective and valued. It changes the focus from current medical management practices that center on the needs of health care organizations and providers to practices that center on patients and health plan members.

■ Conclusion

To identify and manage population-based risk, new information systems, tracking mechanisms, and medical management procedures are necessary. To better manage aggregate costs and unit costs, multidisciplinary care teams must concentrate on the causes of acute care episodes: the underlying psychological, economic, and sociological factors that affect the incidence and prevalence of disease and injuries. Care teams use practice guidelines to identify the least costly and most clinically appropriate settings for direct patient care. This shift in treatment strategy requires that delivery systems take more responsibility for providing care, in three ways:

1. Provide care that best fits the medical, social, and cultural profile of the enrolled population;
2. Maintain and improve the health status of at-risk groups; and
3. Lower the cost of care for individuals and the community.

For MCOs to realize significant long-term savings, a genuine public-private sector partnership is required. All major stakeholders in the health care industry—MCOs, members, employers, practitioners, delivery systems, community organizations, and the government—share a common interest in managing care more effectively by managing risk sooner and better. A partnership approach cuts across the distinctions between for-profit and not-for-profit providers, traditional and complementary medicine, and institutional and alternative settings for care. The improvement of patient care within fixed budgets requires a fundamental redesign of the entire health care delivery system. This is the major challenge for health care reform at the local, state, and federal levels.

Note: This chapter is adapted from the following publications:

■ *The Capitation Sourcebook: A Practical Guide to Managing At-Risk Arrangements,* Chapter 1: The Power and Potential of Capitation. Written by Peter Boland, Ph.D., and published by Boland Healthcare, Inc., Berkeley, CA.

■ *Redesigning Healthcare Delivery: A Practical Guide to Reengineering, Restructuring and Renewal,* Chapter 1: The Role of Reengineering in Healthcare Delivery. Written by Peter Boland, Ph.D., and published by Boland Healthcare, Inc., Berkeley, CA.

■ Key Terms

Business strategy
Buy-in
Change strategy
Comprehensive
   information systems
Core competencies
Cultural change

Eliminate redundancy
Leadership
Managing chronic care
Monitoring high cost/
   high risk
Multidisciplinary teams
Personal care plans

Population-based disease
   management
Reengineering process
Stakeholders
Treatment protocols
Use of new technology
Values

NOTES

1. R. Hamer, "HMO Regional Market Analysis," *InterStudy Competitive Edge,* Vol. 7.1 Part III (July 1997), 1-150.

2. Ibid.

3. Ibid.

4. J. P. Kassirer, "Is Managed Care Here to Stay?" *New England Journal of Medicine,* Vol. 336, No. 14 (April 3, 1997), 1013-1014.

5. R. Hamer, "HMO Industry Trends," *InterStudy Competitive Edge*, Vol. 7.1 Part II (April 1997), 1-113.

6. E. Ginzberg and M. Ostow, "Managed Care—A Look Back and a Look Ahead," *New England Journal of Medicine*, Vol. 336, No. 14 (April 3, 1997), 1018-1020.

7. Hamer, Part III (April 1997).

8. R. Winslow, "Health Care Inflation Revives in Minneapolis Despite Cost-Cutting," *Wall Street Journal* (May 19, 1998), A1, 14.

9. M. Grobman, "Managed Care's Last Frontier," *Business & Health,* Vol. 15, No. 5 (May 1997), 31-34.

10. B. Berlin, "Whither Managed Care?" *New Jersey Medicine,* Vol. 94, No. 5 (May 1997), 27-29.

11. P. W. Nauert, "Managed Care: A Year 2000 Design," *National Underwriter,* Vol. 101, No. 17 (April 28, 1997), 14-17.

12. J. D. DeRosa, "POS Plans May Be the Wave of the Future," *National Underwriter*, Vol. 101, No. 17 (April 28, 1997), 14.

13. Ibid.

14. D. Borfitz, "The MSA Experiment: Controlling Costs by Expanding Patient Choice," *Strategic Health Care Marketing*, Vol. 14, No. 8 (August 1997), 1-4.

15. Ibid.

16. A. Adelson, "Union for Doctors to Join Forces with Government Workers," *New York Times* (August 27, 1997), A18.

17. DeRosa, op. cit.

18. J. Niedzielski, "HMOs Hike Premiums after So-So '96," *National Underwriter* (March 17, 1997), 1.

19. Hamer, Part II (April 1997).

20. J. McGuire, "Aetna Enters Seattle HMO Market with Purchase of VMHP," *Managed Care Outlook,* Vol. 10, No. 16 (August 8, 1997), 3.

21. J. C. Goldsmith, M. J. Goran, and J. G. Nackel, "Managed Care Comes of Age," *Healthcare Forum Journal,* Vol. 38, No. 5 (September/October, 1995), 14-24.

22. M. Brown, "Health Care 2015: Flight of the Butterfly," *Physician Executive,* Vol. 22, No. 1 (January 1996), 5-11.

23. 29 U.S.C. §§1001-1461.

24. *Group Life & Health Insurance Company v. Royal Drug Company,* 440 U.S. 205, 211 (1979).

25. *Union Labor Life Insurance Company v. Pireno,* 458 U.S. 119, 129 (1982).

26. *New York State Conference of Blue Cross & Blue Shield Plans v. Travelers Insurance Company,* 514 U.S. 645 (1995).

27. Administrative Letter 95-10, Virginia Bureau of Insurance, State Corporation Commission (1995). At the time this chapter was written, some VBOI regulators interpreted the Administrative Letter to mean that such arrangements were, in fact, illegal, even if they offered state mandated benefits and complied with form and rate filing requirements.

28. American Academy of Family Physicians, "Gag Clauses in Managed Care Contracts," web page: www.aafp.org/managed/gagrule.html (July 19, 1996).

29. S. 701, 105th Congress, 1st Session (1997).

30. "Managed Care: Explicit Gag Clauses Not Found in HMO Contracts, But Physician Concerns Remain." GAO # HEHS-97-175.

31. *Cigna Healthplan of Louisiana. v. Louisiana,* 82 F.3d 642 (5th Cir. 1996); *Texas Association v. Prudential Insurance Company,* No. 95-50807 (5th Cir. Feb. 14, 1997); *Prudential Insurance Company v. National Park Medical Center,* No. LR-C-95-514, F.Supp. (E.D. Ark. Jan. 31, 1997).

32. Maryland Code, Health-General, §19-710.2.

33. "Compensation Monitor: The Growth of Capitation Continues," *Managed Care* (January, 1997).

34. "Part 5: Payment by Capitation and the Quality of Care," *The New England Journal of Medicine,* Vol. 335, No. 16 (October 17, 1996).

35. California SB 317 (1997).

36. Connecticut SB 1159 (1997).

37. Louisiana S. 724 (signed by Governor, July 9, 1997).

38. 42 C.F.R. §417.479, as published at 61 Fed. Reg. 13430, 13446 (Mar. 27, 1996), as amended at 61 Fed. Reg. 69034, 69049 (Dec. 31, 1996), effective Jan. 1, 1997.

39. 42 USC 1395dd (1985).

40. Florida Stat. Sec. 408.7056 (1985). Code of Virginia, Title 38.2, Chapter 54 (§§ 38.2-5400 through 38.2-5409).

41. Minnesota SF 960 (effective July 1, 1997).

42. G. Anders, "Health Against Wealth," Houghton Mifflin Company, 1996, 22.

43. The Commonwealth Fund, *Patients' Experience with Managed Care: A Survey* (July 1995).

44. Kaiser Family Foundation, *Survey of Americans' Perceptions about For-Profit and Not-for-Profit Health Care* (January 1998).

45. Ibid.

46. Kaiser Family Foundation/Harvard University, *National Survey of Americans' Views on Consumer Protection* (January 1998).

47. "California Task Force Release Managed Care Recommendations: AAHP Urges Careful Assessment," *AAHP in the States* (January 22, 1998), 1.

48. P. Keating, "Why You May Be Getting the Wrong Medicine," *Money* (June 1997). Also see, M. Green, "Pharmaceutical Payola: How Secret Commercial Deals Are Dictating Your Next Prescription and Harming Your Health," A report by Mark Green, Public Advocate for the City of New York (August 1997).

49. B. R. Motheral, "Pharmacy Benefit Management Factors Influencing Utilization and Costs in a Pharmacy Benefit Program," *Drug Benefit Trends* (October 1996).

50. Academy of Managed Care Pharmacy, "A Pharmacist's Guide to Principles and Practices of Managed Care Pharmacy" (Alexandria, Va., 1995).

51. L. Muir, "Disease Management," *Hospital and Health Networks* (June 1997).

52. D. Cassack, "Pharmacy Benefit Management's Second Generation," *The Business and Medicine Report* (July/August 1995).

53. "FDA Regulates Advertising and Marketing of PBMs," *Wall Street Journal* (January 6, 1998).

54. J. Marcille and P. Wynn, "Reinventing the PBM," *Managed Care* (April 1997).

55. "Some HMOs Now Put Doctors on a Budget for Prescription Drugs," *Wall Street Journal* (May 22, 1997).

56. D. S. Mayes, *Managed Dental Care: A Guide to Dental HMOs* (International Foundation of Employee Benefit Plans, 1993).

57. *Health Care Financing Review* (Fall 1996).

58. National Institute of Dental Research, *The National Survey of Oral Health in U.S. Employed Adults and Seniors: 1985-1986* (1987).

59. National Association of Dental Plans, *Dental Market Facts* (March 22, 1997).

60. American Dental Association, *ADA Survey of Dental Practice* (1996).

61. American Dental Association, *ADA Survey of Dental Practice* (1995).

62. American Dental Association, *"A Comparison of Male and Female Dentists: Work Related Issues"* (November 1997).

63. "KPMG Survey of Employer Sponsored Health Benefits, 1991-97," *Employee Benefit Plan Review* (October 1997).

64. M. A. Thompson, M.D., Letter to the Editor, *New England Journal of Medicine*, Vol. 334, No. 16 (April 16, 1996), 1061.

65. M. Mulligan, "Cloudy Picture of Vision Care Coming into Focus For Managed Care Firms," *Managed Care* (July 1995), 25-26.

66. R. A. Berenson, "Beyond Competition," *Health Affairs*, Vol. 16, No. 2 (March/ April 1997), 171-180.

67. J. R. Gabel, "Ten Ways HMOs Have Changed During the 1990s," *Health Affairs*, Vol. 16, No. 3 (May/June, 1997), 134-145.

68. M. R. Gold, et al., "A National Survey of the Arrangements Managed Care Plans Make with Physicians," *New England Journal of Medicine*, Vol. 333, No. 25 (December 21, 1995), 1678-1683.

69. J. C. Robinson and L. P. Casalino, "Vertical Integration and Organizational Networks in Health Care," *Health Affairs*, Vol. 15, No. 1 (Spring 1996), 7-22.

■ Resources

The following Internet sites are recommended sources for additional information:

1. Medicare: http://www.medicare.gov

2. TRICARE: http://www.ha.osd.mel/tricare

3. Medicaid: http://medicaid.apwa.org

4. Legislative information: http://thomas.loc.gov/home/thomas.html

GLOSSARY

A

ACCESS   Right to enter or use health care services.

ACCREDITATION   A designation granted to an organization that meets the eligibility requirements and, when subjected to an evaluation process, demonstrates compliance with the standards of a recognized professional organization.

ACCREDITING BODY   An organization founded for the purposes of setting standards, surveying for compliance with standards, and granting or denying recognition to entities that qualify for and seek such designation.

ADJUSTED AVERAGE PER CAPITA COST (AAPCC)   Health Care Financing Administration's (HCFA) basis of payment to HMOs.

ADJUSTED COMMUNITY RATE (ACR)   Uniform capitation rate charged to all enrollees in a plan based on adjustments for risk factors such as age and gender.

AGENCY FOR HEALTH CARE POLICY AND RESEARCH (AHCPR)   Lead agency (under the U.S. Department of Health and Human Services) charged with supporting research designed to improve the quality of health care, reduce its cost, and broaden access to essential services. Its research programs produce practical, science-based information for use by medical providers, consumers, and health care purchasers.

ANNUITANTS   Term applied to federal employees who retire with Federal Employees Health Benefits coverage.

ANTITRUST LAWS   Laws aimed at the protection of competition.

AUTHORIZATIONS   Consent or endorsement by a primary care physician for patient referral to ancillary services and specialists.

AVERAGE WHOLESALE PRICE (AWP)   Price set by the manufacturer for a drug.

B

BALANCED BUDGET ACT OF 1997 (BBA '97)   A joint resolution to reconcile the budget for fiscal year 1998 (Public Law 105-33). Among numerous provisions, it requires states to grant some regulatory flexibility to risk-assuming provider-sponsored networks for Medicare managed care products; authorizes six sites for a Medicare managed care subvention demonstration between the Health Care Financing Administration (HCFA) and the Department of Defense (DOD); and establishes the Medicare+Choice program.

BENEFIT Amount payable by an insurance company to a claimant, assignee, or beneficiary when the insured suffers a loss covered by the policy.

BUSINESS OF INSURANCE The McCarran-Ferguson Act, passed by Congress in 1945, reserved to the states the regulation of the "business of insurance." The term identifies the traditional boundaries between what the states regulate and what the federal government regulates by the preemptions found in the Employee Retirement Income Security Act (ERISA).

C

CAPITATION Method of payment for health services in which a physician or hospital is paid a fixed amount for each enrollee regardless of the actual number or nature of services provided to each person.

CARVE-OUT Term used to describe certain services offered by an MCO but singled out for individual management, usually with a capitation arrangement. Carve-out services are used for management of chronic diseases; long-term care; mental health, vision, and dental care; and prescription drugs. Also called a specialty managed care arrangement.

CASE MANAGEMENT Planned approach to manage service or treatment to an individual with a serious medical problem. Its dual goal is to contain costs and promote more effective intervention to meet patient needs. Often referred to as large case management.

CLAIM Demand to the insurer by or on behalf of an insured person for the payment of benefits under a policy.

COINSURANCE Portion of incurred medical expenses, usually a fixed percentage, that the patient must pay out of pocket. Usually used in indemnity insurance.

COMMUNITY-RATED Method of developing group-specific capitation rates by a health plan that generally does not account for unique characteristics of the group. The rate is based on the total experience of a given geographic area or "community."

CONSOLIDATED LICENSURE FOR ENTITIES ASSUMING RISK (CLEAR) Health insurance regulatory reform initiative sponsored by the National Association of Insurance Commissioners. When completed, it is designed to create a seamless, even licensure process for all entities assuming risk, no matter what the corporate structure of such entities.

CONSOLIDATED OMNIBUS BUDGET RECONCILIATION ACT (COBRA)
A law that requires employers with group health plans to offer participants and beneficiaries the opportunity to purchase the continuation of health care coverage for a limited period of time after the occurrence of a qualifying event, which is usually the termination of employment. Applies to private employers with 20 or more employees.

CONSUMER ASSESSMENT OF HEALTH PLANS SURVEY (CAHPS)   A standard survey tool to measure both health plan quality and consumer satisfaction.

COORDINATED CARE PLANS   Plans that include health maintenance organizations (HMOs), preferred provider organizations (PPOs), and provider-sponsored organizations (PSOs).

COPAYMENT   A fixed payment (usually $5-10) by the patient paid to the provider at each encounter in managed care. It can also be used as an umbrella term referring to the patient's part of any insured expense: a deductible or a coinsurance payment.

CORPORATE CULTURE   The unique cohesion of values, goals, myths, heroes, styles, and symbols that define the work environment of an organization.

CURRENT MEMBER SURVEY   A type of survey that measures members' satisfaction level with general elements of a plan such as administration, claims, provider services, and benefits.

D

DEDUCTIBLE   Amount of covered expenses that must be incurred and paid by an insured person before benefits become payable by the insurer.

DIRECT LIABILITY   A concept in the law of negligence that holds a person liable for the consequence of his or her own acts.

DISEASE MANAGEMENT PROGRAM   Coordinated efforts of health care professionals focused on a particular disease. Incorporates multiple components, including patient and provider education, medication compliance, guidelines for treatment of the disease, data analysis (includes integration of medical, pharmacy, laboratory, and other data), cognitive services, provider compensation for contributions, patient counseling, and case management services.

DISEASE-SPECIFIC QUESTIONNAIRE   Patient survey tool that measures factors associated with a specific disease.

DRUG UTILIZATION REVIEW (DUR)   The systematic evaluation of physicians' prescribing, pharmacists' dispensing, and patients' use of drugs; also called drug use evaluation (DUE). The goal is to ensure high quality of service to the patient at an affordable cost through appropriate prescribing and use of drugs.

DUAL-ELIGIBLE   Term applied to individuals who qualify to receive benefits under two programs, typically the Medicare and Medicaid programs.

E

ELECTRONIC DATA EXCHANGE (EDI)   The transmission of documents from one computer application to another computer application using a standardized format.

EMERGENCY MEDICAL TREATMENT AND ACTIVE LABOR ACT (EMTALA)   Federal law that requires any hospital with an emergency department to examine all individuals who seek care to determine if an emergency medical condition exists and to stabilize the patient's condition or transfer the patient to another facility for treatment; prohibits the delaying of screening examinations in order to inquire about the method of payment or insurance status.

EMPLOYEE RETIREMENT INCOME SECURITY ACT OF 1974 (ERISA)
A law that mandates reporting and disclosure requirements for group health plans, including MCOs.

EMPLOYER COALITION   The organization of broad-based employers for the purpose of establishing purchasing power within the health care arena.

ENCOUNTER   An in-person meeting between a health plan member and a health care provider during which services are provided. Also used to distinguish between a visit with a capitated provider versus a visit with a provider reimbursed on a fee-for-service basis.

ENROLLEE   Health plan participant, member, or eligible individual in a managed care program.

EVIDENCE-BASED MEDICINE   The systematic selection of clinical processes, based on studies that offer the greatest degree of confidence in their conclusions. The resulting information is compiled into treatment protocols designed to decrease medical costs and maintain or improve health care quality.

210

EXPERIENCE-RATED   Determination of premium or capitation rates for a group risk based wholly or partly on that group's previous cost and utilization experience.

F

FEDERAL ACQUISITION REGULATIONS (FAR)   Codifies uniform policies for acquisition of supplies and services by federal agencies: Department of Defense, General Services Administration, and National Aeronautics and Space Administration. The official FAR appears in the Code of Federal Regulations at 48 CFR Chapter 1.

FEDERAL EMPLOYEES HEALTH BENEFITS PROGRAM (FEHBP)   Federal program providing cost-sharing health benefits to active and retired federal civilian employees and their dependents.

FEE-FOR-SERVICE   Method of payment for provider services based on each visit or service rendered.

FEE SCHEDULE   Maximum dollar or unit allowances for health services that apply under a specific contract.

FORMER MEMBER SURVEY   A type of survey used to determine reasons why a member disenrolled from the plan and that person's overall satisfaction level while a member.

FORMULARY   List of preferred pharmaceutical products, based on evaluations of their efficacy, safety, and cost-effectiveness, that are to be used by a managed care plan's network physicians.

FOUNDATION FOR ACCOUNTABILITY (FACCT)   Private organization, founded in 1995, that assesses how well a plan keeps its members healthy, helps enrollees recover from illness or live with chronic illness, and adapts to the changing needs of its members.

G

GATEKEEPER   Role description of the primary care physician who serves to control utilization and referral of enrollees in HMOs.

GHOSTS   Beneficiaries eligible for Department of Defense-sponsored programs but who choose private health care options for primary coverage.

GROUP-MODEL HMO   HMO staffing that occurs through contracting with multispeciality medical groups to care for plan members. Physicians are not employees of the HMO but are considered as a closed panel.

H

HEADCOUNT REPORT   Report issued by the Office of Personnel Management that provides a count of enrollments by payroll offices for the last payroll paid during the 1st through the 15th of March and September.

HEALTH CARE FINANCING ADMINISTRATION (HCFA)   Branch of the U.S. Department of Health and Human Services charged with oversight and financial management of government-related health care programs such as Medicare and Medicaid.

HEALTH CARE PREPAYMENT PLAN (HCPP)   The HCFA program that allows managed care groups to organize, finance, and deliver Medicare Part B services and be reimbursed for such services on a reasonable cost basis.

HEALTH CONTINUUM MODEL   Programs used by MCOs to better manage all facets of an individual's total health care needs over a period of time.

HEALTH INSURANCE PORTABILITY AND ACCOUNTABILITY ACT (HIPAA)   A 1996 federal law that requires plans to guarantee coverage to any member of an enrolled group, regardless of his or her current or past health status; requires employers with ERISA plans (under the Employee Retirement Income Security Act of 1974) to provide "parity" between mental health and other health benefits; guarantees the right of at least a 48-hour stay for maternity admissions; and authorizes a four-year pilot test of Medical Savings Accounts.

HEALTH INSURANCE PURCHASING COOPERATIVE (HIPC)   Purchasing alliance for small employers to purchase affordable health coverage for their employees and their dependents.

HEALTH MAINTENANCE ORGANIZATION (HMO)   Organization that provides for a wide range of comprehensive health care services for a specified group of enrollees for a fixed, periodic prepayment. There are several models of HMOs, including the staff model, group model, independent practice association, and mixed model.

HEALTH PLAN EMPLOYER DATA AND INFORMATION SET (HEDIS)   A national, standardized method for measuring quality of care, member access, satisfaction, financial stability, and other aspects of MCOs.

HEALTH RISK ASSESSMENTS   Voluntary survey instruments that ask adult members about health-related lifestyles habits, degree of readiness to change lifestyles, and personal preferences for particular activities that reduce health risks.

I

INDEMNITY INSURANCE   Health care insurance plan providing benefits in a predetermined amount for covered services. Traditionally, payment is made on a fee-for-service basis with no involvement by the insurer in the actual delivery of health care services.

INDEPENDENT PRACTICE ASSOCIATION (IPA)   Association of individual physicians that provides services at a negotiated per capita rate, for a flat retainer fee, or on a negotiated fee-for-service basis. It is one model of HMO managed care.

INSURANCE OFFICER   Title of individual responsible for administration of FEHB Program activities at each local agency or federal installation; also referred to as a health benefits officer.

J

JOINT COMMISSION ON ACCREDITATION OF HEALTHCARE ORGANIZATIONS (JCAHO)   Private, voluntary accrediting organization for all types of health care organizations.

L

LEAST EXPENSIVE ALTERNATE TREATMENT (LEAT)   Criteria often used by dental plans to limit their liability to that of the least expensive but professionally acceptable treatment.

M

MAIL SERVICE PHARMACY   Popular program that offers aggressive discounts for prescriptions filled through mail orders; typical service provides a 90-day supply of medication for a single copay and a single dispensing fee.

MANAGED CARE   Term used to describe the coordination of financing and provision of health care to produce high-quality health care on a cost-effective basis.

MANAGED INDEMNITY   Use of utilization controls in traditional fee-for-service health insurance plans in order to reduce cost and inappropriate care.

MANAGEMENT INFORMATION SYSTEMS (MISs)   Term used to describe computer systems that gather, store, and report information as needed. The three most common types are applications reporting systems, database management systems, and decision support systems.

MANDATED BENEFITS   Health care coverage required by state law to be included in health insurance contracts.

MEDICAID   State programs with federal matching funds for public health assistance to persons, regardless of age, whose income and resources are insufficient to pay for health care.

MEDICAL NECESSITY   Term used by insurers to describe medical treatment that is appropriate and rendered in accordance with generally accepted standards of medical practice.

MEDICAL SAVINGS ACCOUNTS (MSAs)   A form of indemnity insurance that combines a high-deductible policy with a savings account. The savings from a higher deductible is deposited in a medical savings account to cover routine medical expenses, a high-deductible insurance plan covers expenses that exceed the deductible, and, at year-end, the consumer keeps any remaining balance in the account.

MEDICARE   Federally sponsored program under the Social Security Act that provides hospital benefits, supplementary medical care, and catastrophic coverage to persons 65 years of age and older and some younger persons who are covered under Social Security benefits.

MEDICARE+CHOICE   New Medicare Part C program established by the Balanced Budget Act of 1997 (BBA '97). The law creates a new authority that permits contracts between the Health Care Financing Administration (HCFA) and a variety of different managed care and fee-for-service entities, including coordinated care plans; religious, fraternal benefit society plans; and private fee-for-service plans.

MEMBER   A subscriber or eligible dependent in a health plan.

MEMBER MONTHS   The average number of members for the period times the number of months in the period. It is calculated by summing the number of members for each month in the period.

214

MILITARY HEALTH SERVICES SYSTEM (MHSS) Federal health benefits program for active duty military personnel, retirees, their dependents, and survivors.

MILITARY TREATMENT FACILITY (MTF) Hospitals and clinics operated worldwide by the Army, Navy, and Air Force.

MULTIPLE EMPLOYER WELFARE ARRANGEMENTS (MEWAs)/MULTIPLE EMPLOYER TRUSTS (METs) Groups of small employers that join together (by nature of their business or regional location) to offer co-developed health benefit plans to their employees.

MULTISPECIALTY GROUP PRACTICE Independent physicians' group that organizes or is organized to contract with a managed care plan to provide medical services to enrollees. The physicians are not employees of the HMO, but are employed by the group practice.

N

NATIONAL ASSOCIATION OF INSURANCE COMMISSIONERS (NAIC) National organization of state officials charged with regulating insurance. It has no official power but wields tremendous influence. The association was formed to promote national uniformity in insurance regulations.

NATIONAL COMMITTEE FOR QUALITY ASSURANCE (NCQA) Private, voluntary accrediting organization for managed care. It assesses quality, credentialing, utilization management, customer rights, preventive health services, and medical records. Developed and oversees the Health Plan Employer Data and Information Set (HEDIS).

NEGLIGENCE A body of law that assigns legal responsibility to a party as a result of his or her acts or omissions, usually by the payment of money damages to the injured party.

NEGOTIATED FEES Managed care plans and providers mutually agree on a set fee for each service. This negotiated rate is usually based on services defined by the Current Procedural Terminology (CPT) codes, generally at a discount from what the provider would usually charge. Providers cannot charge more than this fee.

NETWORK-MODEL HMO Provider arrangements that contract with a number of independent practice associations (IPAs) or group practices to provide physician services to HMO enrollees. This model is a multiple provider arrangement that can be either an open or closed panel.

NETWORK PROVIDERS Limited grouping or panel of providers in a managed care arrangement with several delivery points. Enrollees may be required to use only network providers or may have financing liability for using non-network providers for medical services.

NON-NETWORK PROVIDERS Non-contracted or unapproved health providers who are outside a managed care arrangement.

O

OPEN-ENDED HMO Hybrid HMO product that allows members to use physicians outside the plan in exchange for additional personal liability in the form of a deductible, coinsurance, or copayment.

OPEN-ENROLLMENT PERIOD The period of time agreed to by an employer and a health plan for all employees to review their health care options and elect to make any changes for the forthcoming year. Usually done 30 to 60 days prior to the employer's renewal date with the health plan.

OUTCOME MEASUREMENT Tool used to assess a health system's or provider's performance that measures the results of a given intervention or course of treatments.

OUT-OF-NETWORK CARE Medical services obtained by managed care plan members from unaffiliated or non-contracted health care providers. In many plans, such care will not be reimbursed unless previous authorization for such care is obtained.

OUT-OF-POCKET EXPENSES Those health care costs that must be borne by the insured because they are not covered under an insurance contract.

OVERUTILIZATION Term used to describe inappropriate or excessive use of medical services that add to health care costs.

P

PER DIEM Literally, per day. Term that is applied to determining costs for a day of care and is an average that does not reflect true cost for each patient.

PER MEMBER PER MONTH (PMPM) Computational designation for each enrollee in a managed care program. It is commonly abbreviated as PMPM.

PHARMACY AND THERAPEUTICS (P&T) COMMITTEE Health plan committee typically composed of physicians, pharmacists, and other health care personnel. The committee selects pharmaceuticals for inclusion in the prescription drug formulary that are the most appropriate, rational, and affordable products for use; recommends guidelines for appropriate use of medications; and develops policies for the evaluation, selection, and therapeutic use of pharmaceuticals.

PHARMACY BENEFIT MANAGEMENT COMPANY   Organization under contract with an MCO to provide drug benefit services, including formulary management, rebates, discounted pharmacy networks, mail service pharmacies, and electronic claims processing.

PHYSICIAN-HOSPITAL ORGANIZATION (PHO)   Group practice arrangement that occurs when hospitals and physicians organize for purposes of contracting with managed care organizations. These relationships are formally organized, contractual, or corporate in character and include physicians outside the boundaries of a hospital's medical staff.

POINT-OF-SERVICE (POS) PLANS   Combination of HMO and PPO features. They provide a comprehensive set of health benefits and offer a full range of health services much the same as the HMO. However, the members do not have to choose how to receive services until they need them. The member can then opt to use the defined managed care program, or can go out-of-plan for services but pay the difference for non-plan benefits (e.g., 100 percent coverage for managed care vs. 80 percent coverage out-of-plan).

PRACTICE GUIDELINES   Specific, evidence-based recommendations to standardize clinical processes for a diagnosis and treatment of a disease or illness; designed to achieve consistent, favorable outcomes.

PRACTICE MANAGEMENT COMPANY   A company that manages all business aspects of a provider's practice. The company may purchase all or a portion of a practice and employ the providers or may contract to manage the practice for a fee.

PREAUTHORIZATION   Previous approval for specialist referral or non-emergency health care services.

PREEMPTION   The negation of the effect of one law by another such as in the case of ERISA preemption.

PREFERRED PROVIDER ORGANIZATION (PPO)   Managed care arrangement consisting of a group of hospitals, physicians, and other providers who have contracts with an insurer, employer, third-party administrator, or other sponsoring group to provide health care services to covered persons.

PREMIUM   Periodic payment to keep an insurance policy in force.

PRIMARY CARE PHYSICIAN (PCP)   Primary deliverer and manager of health care, central to controlling costs and utilization. The PCP provides basic care to the enrollee, initiates referrals to specialists, and provides follow-up care. Refers exclusively to other contracted providers and admits patients only to contracted hospitals. Usually defined as a physician practicing in such areas as internal medicine, family practice, and pediatrics.

PRIVATE FEE-FOR-SERVICE PLANS   Health plans that reimburse providers on a fee-for-service basis and are authorized to charge enrolled beneficiaries up to 115 percent of the plan's payment schedule (which may differ from the Medicare fee schedule).

PROFILES   Systematic method of collecting, collating, and analyzing patient data to create a summary of distinctive features or characteristics of the medical practice for a provider or for the collective practice of providers in a health plan. Also used to depict a patient's medical status.

PROSPECTIVE REVIEW   Data-gathering technique that uses projected figures or current data to determine future costs or services.

PROVIDERS   Term used to describe medical professionals and service organizations that provide health care services.

PROVIDER-SPONSORED ORGANIZATION (PSO)   Public or private entity established by health care providers that provides a substantial proportion of health care items and services directly through affiliated providers who share, directly or indirectly, substantial financial risk.

Q

QUALITY IMPROVEMENT   Formal set of activities designed to monitor, evaluate, and improve the key administrative and clinical processes of an organization.

QUALITY OF LIFE ASSESSMENTS   Questionnaires designed to capture information about health-related quality of life; divided into general health and disease-specific categories. The best known is the Short Form 36 Health Survey developed by John Ware.

R

RATING   The process of developing an appropriate premium price for a group or population to be insured.

REENGINEERING Methodology to structure work processes based on organizational purpose and performance, with the goals of work simplification, improved job skills, better motivation of performance, and the provision of necessary equipment, technology, and facility support.

REFERRAL Primary care physician-directed transfer of a patient to a specialty physician or specialty care.

RETENTION Activities within the sales and marketing departments to ensure that current members remain with the plan at renewal.

RIDER A document that modifies or amends an insurance contract. Also called a supplemental benefit. Often used to refer to pharmacy, mental health, vision, and dental coverage.

RISK Chance of incurring financial loss by an insurer or provider.

RISK-BASED CAPITAL (RBC) Concept used to assess the solvency of insurance companies. An RBC formula establishes a minimum amount of capital required to absorb the potential risks to which an insurance company is exposed.

RISK SHARING Apportionment of chance of incurring financial loss by insurers, managed care organizations, and health care providers.

S

SELF-INSURERS Employers, businesses, and other entities that choose to assume the responsibilities of an insurance company to insure their beneficiaries.

SERVICE AREA The defined, geographical location where an MCO can offer services based on provider availability.

SERVICE AREA WAIVER An exemption that allows MCOs to enroll members who reside outside their defined service area. The waiver also defines the requirements for the member to be enrolled in the plan.

SMALL-AREA VARIATION ANALYSIS Method developed by John Wennberg, M.D., at Dartmouth College, to identify differences in the utilization of health services (by disease category and within a limited geographic area) through the analysis of claims data.

SOCIAL SECURITY ACT Law under which the federal government operates the Old Age, Survivors, Disability, and Health Insurance (OASDHI) Program. Includes Medicare and Medicaid.

STAFF-MODEL HMO   HMO that owns the clinical facilities used by patients enrolled in the HMO. The physicians providing service are directly employed by the HMO and they provide service only to patients enrolled in the HMO plan.

STAKEHOLDERS   Those with a stake in the cost and quality of health care services, including patients, employers, providers, communities, and government.

T

TAFT-HARTLEY TRUSTS   The Labor Management Relations Act of 1947 (Taft-Hartley Act), provided for the establishment of trusts to offer health benefits to employees whose benefits are collectively bargained.

THERAPEUTIC INTERCHANGE   Approved replacement of an originally prescribed drug by one that is equivalent in terms of effectiveness and results, as determined in advance by a panel of physicians.

THIRD-PARTY ADMINISTRATOR (TPA)   Method by which an outside person or firm, not a party to a contract, maintains all records regarding the persons covered by an insurance plan. A TPA may also pay claims.

TORT   A wrong for which the law will hold the actor responsible. Torts may be intentional (e.g., assault or defamation), or unintentional (e.g., negligence).

TOTAL QUALITY MANAGEMENT (TQM)   Systematic, mission-, and value-based approach to continuously monitor and improve an organization's key business and clinical processes to achieve better results. Also referred to as continuous quality improvement (CQI).

TRICARE   Nationwide Department of Defense (DOD) managed care program, operated in partnership with civilian contractors, that is designed to ensure high-quality consistent health care benefits; preserve beneficiaries' choice of health care providers; improve access to care; and contain health care costs. Program offers a choice of a health maintenance organization, a preferred provider organization, or a fee-for-service program (the former CHAMPUS program).

U

USUAL, CUSTOMARY, AND REASONABLE (UCR) FEES   Charges of health care providers that are consistent with charges from similar providers for identical or similar services in a given locale.

W

WAIVERS   Term usually associated with the Medicare or Medicaid programs by which the government waives certain regulations or rules for a managed care or insurance program to operate in a certain geographic area.

WELLNESS PROGRAMS   Intervention strategies designed to improve health and prevent disease that are sponsored by employers or managed care organizations, typically in coordination with employers.

WITHHOLD ARRANGEMENTS   Portion of a provider's salary, fees, or capitation that is held back until performance in relation to quality and utilization is examined at the end of each year. If performance was at least satisfactory, withholds are released to the provider.

INDEX